SURVIVAL
AFTER 55

God Bless You
Vada Lee Barkley

By
Vada Lee Barkley

Phil. 4:13

RANDALL HOUSE PUBLICATIONS
P.O. BOX 17306
NASHVILLE, TN 37217

SURVIVE AND THRIVE AFTER 55

© Copyright 1987
Randall House Publications
Nashville, Tennessee
ISBN 0-89265-130-X

All rights in this book are reserved. No part of the text may be reproduced in any manner without permission in writing from the publisher except in the case of brief quotations for purposes of a review.

Printed in the United States of America

Editor's Preface

Seldom does one find a book with such a wealth of vital information on the aging process and retirement considerations. Properly placed priorities insist on the reading of this book in one's fifties, at least. For those who have passed this milestone, its reading is a must.

Vada Lee Barkley, nearing three score and ten years herself, with sparkle and wit, reveals the vibrance and vitality one may exude in the golden years. *Survive and Thrive After 55* is a strong testimony to the productive potential of senior years.

She writes with clarity and conviction from personal experience, painstaking research, and concern for senior citizens. *Survive and Thrive After 55* reveals a person of Christian character, competence, and compassion.

You will enjoy this grand tour through Golden Acres and use this valuable resource tool again and again. Happy reading!

Harrold D. Harrison
Editor-In-Chief
Randall House Publications

Table of Contents

Page

Editor's Preface
Foreward
Introduction 1
Chapter:
  1. Welcome to Golden Acres 5
  2. Main Street: Chamber of Commerce 8
  3. Camelot Court: Department of Public Safety 14
  4. Bella Vista Boulevard: Behavioral Sciences
     Center 31
  5. Blue Ridge Heights: Marriage and Family
     Arena 52
  6. Church Avenue: Spiritual Development 68
  7. Commerce Drive: Money Management
     Resources 75
  8. Crestview Development: Housing Facilities 98
  9. Bel-Aire Circle: Physical Health Facilities 110
 10. Sunset Parkway: Golden Acres Mortuary 128
 11. Fairmont Freeway: Residential Section 133
 12. Golden Acres Public Library 137

Foreward

I have known the author of this welcome book, *Survive and Thrive After 55*, for almost forty years. During this time she has approached life's circumstances both pleasant and unpleasant with a positive attitude and a wholesome response which has won for her many friends and enabled her to minister to unnumbered persons.

She has a first-hand knowledge of the trauma of retirement. Through careful research she has discovered ways to reduce the anxiety of this stage of life, and she has given us the benefit of her labors in this helpful manuscript. An English teacher for many years, she fashions her counsel in ways that are creative and intriguing.

Almost every problem confronting retired persons is here addressed—be they the simple challenges or the more complex ones. The reader will find helpful suggestions from selecting the best place to live, to investing funds, to pre-need funeral arrangements.

This book should be read by everyone who is retired, and by those who are approaching retirement during the next decade. One will not only be better informed for the reading, but will have a fun-time doing it.

—John A. Knight
March, 1987

Introduction

When my husband and I drive through the Ozarks, we admire the beautiful homes on top of the mountains.

"Oh, look, Honey!" I'm actually hoping he won't. Negotiating those curves demands undivided attention. "How'd you like to live up there? We could revel in this beauty all year."

Lots of us would relish the scenery. Few, however, are able to afford such luxury. For that lovely home overlooking the gorgeous view didn't just happen.

Think of the struggle
>to clear a road and building site,
>>to dig a well,
>>>to put in a septic tank,
>>>>to haul building materials up the steep grade,
>>>>>to install electricity,
>>>>>>to deliver furniture.

Imagine the cost!

Suppose we look in on the retired owners.

It's after dinner their first night in their new home. The husband opens the drapes. His wife joins him at the picture window. They gaze upon breath-taking scenery under a moonlit sky.

"Honey, we finally made it." He slips an arm around her. "Ever since I used to hunt in the mountains, I've claimed this one. I've always dreamed of living right on top. Now here we are."

"You've always been a dreamer, Dear," she says. "And I love you for that."

"It took a lot of hard work and money, but it's worth it."

The Old Testament character Caleb must have felt like that his first night on top of his mountain. The picture is blurred after nearly forty centuries, but I'll try to explain.

Wiping the remains of his wife's barbequed wild goat

from his mustache, Caleb steps outside his tent. He draws a deep breath, filling his lungs with the invigorating air. He feasts his eyes on the valleys and other mountains around Hebron silhouetted against the sky.

His son-in-law, General Othniel, saunters over from the adjoining tent. Mrs. Caleb and Achsah bring sheepskin mats. Lying there under the stars, Caleb begins to reminisce.

"When I was forty, Othniel, I came to this country with a delegation Moses sent to spy out the land. On that trip God gave me a vision of what He planned for His people. He even promised me this mountain," Caleb said. Othniel yawns. He's heard this before.

"Ten spies reported that this was indeed a land of opportunity. 'But,' they told Moses, 'we can't possibly take that country. Why, there are giants everywhere. We look like grasshoppers by the side of them.'

"Only Joshua and I insisted that, with God's help, we could drive out the giants and claim the land. We even carried a huge cluster of grapes between us to tempt the multitude.

"The ten negative reports, however, put fear in the hearts of the Israelis. Instead of obeying God and claiming His promise, they turned back into the wilderness. God decreed that every adult except Joshua and me would die there.

"I wholly followed the Lord. And Moses agreed that God had promised this place to me and my descendants.

"Years later, Joshua led Israel into the Promised Land. When he divided the territory among the tribes, I asked for this mountain. I had to admit that I was 85 years old. But I assured him that the Lord had kept me well and I was as strong as ever. More than anything else, I wanted to realize the dream God had given me.

"Joshua didn't have to remind me. I knew that the sons of Anak, who lived on this mountain, were the biggest and toughest in Canaan. But I had God's promise.

"It hasn't been easy. Sometimes I've had to call on

younger men like you for help. But you didn't mind as long as I gave you my daughter," he chuckled.

"God's been good to me. He's helped me defeat all the giants on my mountain. And if Anak has any more grandsons around here, I'm ready to tackle them."

I'll admit that Caleb probably lived longer than we will live. Our doctors keep coming up with all these diseases, and we have to have them. The trouble with a lot of these new medical treatments is that they have side effects—like bankruptcy.

Assuming Caleb lived as long as Joshua—110 years—we can expect about the same number of years after our retirement. How much of that twenty-five years it took for him to drive out his enemies, the Bible doesn't say. Evidently he spent a lot of that time fighting.

A man of lesser courage would have tottered up to where Joshua was standing and mumbled this request: "As you know, Sir, when I was forty, God promised me that mountain. But I don't know about that now. I've been fighting hard these forty-five years. Part of that time to survive in the wilderness, the rest helping God's people defeat enemies and get settled in this country. I'm about worn out. I'd like to retire now and take life easy. All I ask is a safe place for my tent down here where I can look up at the mountain every day for the rest of my life." Really, now, could you blame him?

But Caleb was no grasshopper. He was a spiritual giant. He never forgot God's plan for him. He refused to take it easy until he "expelled thence the three sons of Anak" (Judges 1:20).

What a model for any retiree! By "retiree" I mean anyone aged 55 or above, not working full time.

"I don't think it's ever God's will for anyone to retire," a lawyer said to a doctor. "Have you ever noticed how often a person dies right after he retires?"

Indeed, haven't we all noticed? In fact, the lawyer merely echoed a popular myth. Based on faulty reasoning—called *non sequitur*—the myth assumes that because a worker retired, he died. Maybe he retired because of illness.

False logic may win court cases. But we need facts to make wise decisions relative to our lives. The truth is, unless forced to retire because of ill health, a worker has a better chance to live longer and enjoy life more by slowing his pace and changing his focus.

Of course, retirement is not for everybody. But if I find God's will for me is to retire, I know He has a plan for my future. That mountain He promised looms ahead. He will help me drive out the giants on my way to the top. I learned a long time ago that if I can't handle a giant, He can.

Who knows? We may have twenty-five years to conquer them and take the mountain.

Chapter 1
Welcome to Golden Acres

Hi, I'm your hostess on Golden Acres Educational Tours. Welcome aboard! My credentials? Come with me back to the day when I joined this growing community.

I've looked forward to my special day. Now that it has come, I wonder if I'm really ready for it.

I've spent hours cleaning out my desk and files. I've lugged that last box to the car. I glance at the hall clock again. It's time for the party.

I saunter into the conference room. I've gone there hundreds of times. But this is different. Today I'm the center of attraction. This is my party. Yet I feel "out of it."

I smile as I greet colleagues. I stare at the gorgeous table. Linen cloth, punch bowl, cups, silverware, dainty napkins imprinted with my name, the cake. Ah, the cake! Edged in candied red roses, it covers a third of the big table. At least it looks that large. The words "Happy Retirement" followed by my first name leap out at me from a frothy bed of icing.

A twinge of nostalgia sweeps over me, like, "I miss you already and I'm not even gone." I wipe a tear before it drops on the cake I'm posed to cut.

I sit as I nibble my cake and sip my punch. Somehow I feel safer sitting.

I relish the farewell remarks of colleagues. I revel in the strokes as the boss speaks. (If only I'd got more of them sooner.) Hands trembling, legs unsteady, I step forward to receive my plaque in appreciation for years of outstanding, dedicated service to the institution. I swallow a lump and respond in an unfamiliar voice—a bit too loud, too fast.

The party ends. I trudge to my car. Inside, I keep hearing: "I'll miss you"; "I envy you"; "Good luck." Before turning the key, I take a long look at the familiar college buildings, my second home.

Whatever else the site represents, it has been a source of security:
>a job
>>friends
>>>a need to fulfill
>>>>a schedule to meet
>>>>>something to look forward to
>>>>>>a sense of worth
>>>>>>>an income.

As I drive away, I leave all those taken-for-granted benefits behind. Tomorrow I must meet a new challenge.

I brace myself and start home.

For me and 5,000 fellow Americans, it's the last day on the job.

After two or three weeks, maybe months, of doing my own thing:
>Sleeping in
>>Reading
>>>Fishing
>>>>Golfing
>>>>>Traveling,

I wonder how I can stand very many years of retirement. To paraphrase the Patriarch Job, "If I retire, shall I live again?"

I make that decision. Unless in the grip of a terminal illness at retirement, I have a choice. I can lie down and die in sight of my dream or get up and do something toward achieving it. I can take my mountain.

What I can do, by God's grace, I will do.

For me, tomorrow has come. I'm so excited about the challenge that I've become a tour guide to share my enthusiasm.

Before we start, I want to give you a brief over-view of our tour.

First, we'll stop at the Chamber of Commerce office on Main Street for orientation into our community. Then, on Camelot Court, we'll visit the Department of Public Safety for safety and crime prevention tips.

On Bella Vista Boulevard we'll see our Behavioral Sciences Center. There we'll gain insight into attitudes and activities that will help us adjust to retirement. The Marriage and Family Arena on Blue Ridge Heights will provide information on how to cope with changing relationships.

At the Cathedral on Church Avenue, we'll participate in a worship service and learn about the senior citizens' program and facilities.

From the church, we'll head for Commerce Drive for a visit with a banker, an attorney, and an automobile dealer. In Golden Acres Housing Development, we'll learn about the housing possibilities for senior adults.

Our lunch stop will be Bel-Aire Circle. As we eat at the hospital cafeteria, a dietitian will talk with us about special nutritional needs of senior adults. In the adjoining clinic, we'll hear about the physical side of the aging process and how to cope with it. In the gym, we'll learn about our physical fitness requirements. Finally, we'll visit a nursing home, where a small percent of our elderly live.

We'll stop by the funeral home on Sunset Parkway to discuss prearranged plans that can save survivors expense and anxiety.

Our return trip promises to be especially thrilling. In a residential section on Fairmont Freeway, we'll meet some of my vivacious neighbors—if we can catch them at home.

Each site we visit will provide basic information on how to make the most of Golden Acres' living. Our final stop, the public library, contains sources of additional information of interest to you.

Everybody ready? Let's go.

Chapter 2
Main Street: Chamber of Commerce

Before the twentieth century, old age, as we know it, did not exist. Sixty years ago, "The average man worked seventy hours a week and died at age forty. Now, a person works forty hours a week and lives to age seventy."[1]

More than 150,000 Americans retire every month. An overwhelming majority of them have a dozen or so years of productive life to enjoy. Robert N. Butler, gerontologist and research psychiatrist at the Washington School of Psychiatry, Washington, D.C., says that by the year 2000 the average man will have twenty-five years of retirement. At the time of his prediction (1975), the average man left the work force at age fifty-seven.[2] It's more like fifty-five now.

The more thoroughly we plan for retirement, the more likely we will be to enjoy it. Retiring *to* something rather than *from* something brings greater satisfaction.

Ideally, planning should begin early, say mid forties. But it's never too late to plan.

Dr. Gaston Foote tells the following story:

A farmer needed a hired hand. One man he interviewed kept saying, "I can always sleep on a stormy night." The farmer thought that statement was strange, but in other respects the man seemed normal. So the farmer hired him.

One night the farmer awoke to the rumbling of thunder and the flash of lightning. Jumping out of bed, he put on his trousers and shoes and dashed down the hall to the hired man's room. Above the sound of roaring thunder and howling wind, he heard snores. A flash of lightning showed a calm face and relaxed body, oblivious to the threatening storm.

Then he remembered the words, "I can always sleep on a stormy night." He went outside to check on things himself. He heard no squawking in the chicken house; he found the door closed. At the barn he found his horses and cattle safely bedded down inside closed stalls. At the hog pen he saw the sows and pigs sleeping peacefully on their favorite mud mattress. He found hay stacks tied down and storage barns secured.

Back in his warm, cozy bed, he drifted off to sleep.[3]

A recent Harris poll reveals that a majority of people agree on seven important steps in preparing for later life:
1. Ensure medical care is available.
2. Prepare a will.
3. Build up savings.
4. Learn about pensions and Social Security benefits.
5. Buy your own home.
6. Develop hobbies, leisure-time activities.
7. Decide whether you want to move or stay where you are.

One-third of those responding said it was important to plan for a new part-time or full-time job.[4]

Whether you're prepared or not, the die is cast. Possibly twenty-five to thirty percent of your life lies ahead. What you do with it is up to you.

Sociologist Robert Atchley found that most married men, especially semiskilled, unskilled, or service men, look forward to retirement. Afterward, however, many object to doing household chores. They may experience conflict or guilt. And they often irritate their wives.

More than half the wives in one survey regretted their husbands' retirement.[5] As Margaret Mead observed: "You have half as much income and twice as much husband."

According to Atchley, women—those among blue-collar, low income, poorly educated, or in ill health in particular—have more trouble than men adjusting to retirement.[6]

"Dread of retirement," Atchley concludes, "is closely related to anticipated financial insecurity. Acceptance of retirement is closely related to having achieved one's job-related goals."[7]

At age sixty-two I retired from full-time work. Someone else assumed my office, my title, and my classes. Most of them, that is. I dumped committee work, administrative responsibilities, most lesson preparation and paper grading. I continued to teach a class or two per semester. For three years I enjoyed the best of both worlds. At sixty-five I retired, a victim of paper-grading burnout. Gradual retirement worked well for me.

The final stage in family life cycles begins with retirement. At that time we face important, often disruptive adjustments:
1. Adjusting to a reduced income
2. Adjusting to retirement
3. Adjusting to a possible move
4. Adjusting to the idea of our death and death of our spouse
5. Adjusting to and coping with a rapidly changing society
6. Maintaining a satisfactory sexual relationship
7. Finding new friends because old friends have died or moved away
8. Adjusting to the decline in physical strength and, in many cases, chronic illness of self or spouse
9. Adjusting to great-grandparenthood.[8]

Atchley outlines the following "Phases of Retirement":

I. Preretirement—in which people "begin to gear themselves for separation from their jobs and the social situations within which they carried out those jobs" and later "develop fairly detailed fantasies of what they think their retirement will be like."

II. Honeymoon—in which people live out the preretirement fantasy. The length of the honeymoon varies.

III. Disenchantment—when the retiree must face reality. The more unrealistic the preretirement fantasy, the more likely we will be to experience disenchantment, even depression. It's depressing to have to start over again to restructure life in retirement.

IV. Reorientation—This is a time for "a realistic view

of alternatives," for exploring new avenues of involvement. Senior Citizens' groups and family and friends can help.

Many retirees omit Phases III and IV.

V. Stability—The retiree becomes self-sufficient, going his own way, managing his own affairs. He now has a "well-developed set of criteria for making choices." Life has become predictable and satisfying.

VI. Termination—In this phase, the retiree assumes the sick and disabled role. He loses his independence and gradually gives up the retirement role, completely losing the dignity of his retirement role when he must enter an institution.[9]

Our greatest challenge as retirees is prolonging Phases I through V and postponing Phase VI. Most of us prefer getting old to the only alternative. Yet we don't want to get old before our time, nor to live too long. We're like the lady who said, "My husband and I don't want to go to a nursing home. We just hope we're killed in a car accident on the way home from a ski trip when we're in our 90's."

We coin euphemisms: Golden Agers, Senior Citizens, Retirees—anything to improve our self-image.

We readily admit our eligibility for a Senior Citizens' discount at the pharmacy, restaurant, or grocery store. Our Golden Agers' pass gets us into national parks. We like that. We proudly show our AARP membership card in exchange for a ten-to-fifteen percent reduction on car rental or motel rates. Yet we resist getting old. Others age; we don't.

A few nights after my husband's sixty-fifth birthday, we attended a Fourth of July celebration. We passed a choice section of chairs reserved for Senior Citizens. Half way through the performance, when our backs hurt so badly we could hardly sit on the bleachers, it dawned on me. We could have sat in those comfortable seats.

According to Census Bureau statistics, the number of Americans age 65 and over has doubled in the past thirty years. The Congressional Office of Technology Assessment announced (October, 1984) that for the first time, people over 65 outnumber teen-agers in the United States. The report predicts that by the year 2010, the number of people over 65 will increase from 26 million to 39.3 million—to almost 14 percent of the population. Within the next fifty years that figure could amount to one-fifth of the nation's population.[10] One person out of five!

Columnist James J. Kilpatrick voiced the concern of us all: "What kind of life will these old folks live?"[11]

While behavioral scientists and politicians wrestle with that question, we senior citizens can do much to determine the answer for ourselves. We haven't lived all these years for nothing. We simply refuse to panic. We've built up enough resilience in our three-score-plus years to assure us that the God who has taken us through those years will see us through the future.

First, we attack certain myths. Butler lists six common ones:

1. The myth of "Aging"
2. The myth of Unproductivity
3. The myth of Disengagement
4. The myth of Inflexibility
5. The myth of Senility
6. The myth of Serenity.[12]

Dispelling these myths strips the specter, Old Age, of its mask. We recognize the phantom as only our shadow. Harmless, if not attractive.

Second, having faced the enemy and found that "he is us," we're free to make friends with him and improve his image. We're amazed that so many famous people have co-existed successfully with him.

At age 73, Colonel Sanders made his first million. He retired as a gas station operator. With his first Social Security check, he invested in Kentucky Fried Chicken.

News anchormen Walter Kronkite and Harry Reasoner have made special documentaries past their retirement age.

Comedians Bob Hope and George Burns continue to entertain. George Burns is 90. Duke Ellington kept up a hectic concert schedule in his 70's. Arthur Fiedler directed his famous Boston Pops orchestra until age 85.

Three of the last four Soviet leaders were in their later years. Golda Meir was Prime Minister during her 70's. Our own President Ronald Reagan, in his 70's, keeps up a hectic pace.

Recently we heard Dr. Norman Vincent Peale preach on TV. He's in his 80's.

The list is endless. In addition to famous people, each of us could name scores of acquaintances who remain active well into their 80's or even 90's. If they can, so can we. We'll talk about them later.

Chapter 3
Camelot Court: Department of Public Safety

Unfortunately, residents of this area are especially vulnerable to crime. On the plus side, however, keeping informed and alert will greatly decrease your chances of becoming a victim.

Here are a few suggestions:

Outside the Home

1. Avoid walking alone at night.
2. If you must walk, stay near other people and be alert for suspicious characters near you.
3. Don't wear expensive clothing or jewelry.
4. Guard your purse. Keep it tucked tightly under your arm. A dangling purse makes an easy target for a snatcher.
5. When making a credit card purchase, check slips before signing them, make sure the clerk returns *your* card, and don't let anyone looking over your shoulder memorize your card as you sign it.
6. After charging an item, ask for the carbon paper and destroy it.
7. Put your money and billfold away before leaving the checkout counter.
8. Don't carry more packages than you can safely manage.
9. Lock your packages in the trunk of the car.
10. Keep your car in good working condition. Check tires before you leave home.
11. Keep your car doors locked and windows closed.
12. Put your purse out of sight.
13. At night, wear a man's hat.

14. If you see a stalled car beside the road, stop at the next lighted telephone booth and call police.
15. Carry a "Please Call Police" sign in your glove compartment. In case of trouble, stick this luminous sign on the back window. Then get back into the car and lock the doors until help comes. A would-be criminal will think the police may be on the way.
16. If you suspect someone is following you, drive to a well-lighted, populated area—a store, a restaurant, or police station—and notify the police. Whatever you do, don't go home.
17. Park in a well-lighted area.
18. Look around before leaving your car.
19. When walking toward your car, be alert.
20. Have your keys ready.
21. Check the back seat before getting into your car.
22. Don't hesitate to make a scene.

Inside the Home

More rapes occur in the home than anywhere else. To lessen your chances of rape or burglary, you can take a number of precautionary measures.
1. Have police make a security check of your home.
2. Install dead bolt locks. According to insurance agents, burglars are 85 percent less likely to break into a house with dead bolt locks. They know anything they steal must go through a window.
3. Leave a key in a dead bolt lock when you're in the house in case of fire. Take the key when you leave.
4. Keep your doors locked. Even if you've just come inside and you're going back out in a minute.
5. Don't open your door to a stranger, especially if you're alone.
6. Invest in adequate outdoor lighting and a peephole.
7. Verify all unexpected repairmen or anyone posing as a representative of a utility company. A reliable employee will not object to your calling his or her

company's business office.
8. Use only initials on mailbox and in telephone directories.
9. If you move, insist on new locks.
10. Keep window blinds closed at night.
11. Be wary of telephone callers who refuse to identify themselves. Don't tell them you're alone.
12. Don't talk to an obscene or nuisance caller. Hang up, gently but firmly.
13. If such calls persist, call your telephone company and/or police.
14. Leave a light on somewhere in the house.
15. Don't hesitate to call police to report suspicious activity.

On Vacation

1. Ask the post office to hold your mail or arrange for someone to pick it up.
2. Stop delivery of your newspaper or ask a neighbor to pick it up.
3. During the summer, arrange to have your lawn mowed.
4. Invest in a timer to turn lights on in different places at specific times.
5. Let your neighbors and police know you're gone.

Our neighbors, Jack and Wanda, look after things for us when we're on a vacation. And we check on their place when they're gone.

One day while they were away, my husband was working in our front yard. Suddenly he saw their garage door go up. He assumed their son's wife was there. But he didn't see a car. Another neighbor came over and the two tried the doors. Finally I called their son's wife, and their son came over to check through the house. No one had been inside. What caused the automatic garage door opener to function on its own remains a mystery. But the good feeling that neighbors are watching makes everyone more comfortable.

Following just two of those suggestions prevented my becoming a victim one afternoon. I'll never forget that nightmare.

I take safety precautions seriously after dark. But in the daytime? Nobody ever gets followed in the daytime. Right? Wrong.

At four o'clock one afternoon, I was cruising down the interstate toward home. Completely relaxed, I was thinking of school and what I had to do the next day. I vaguely remember passing an old battered delivery truck a few miles before leaving the highway.

To avoid traffic and lights, I took a back route. Usually I drove through a park near the lake. Slowing for a rough railroad crossing—I was driving a new car—I saw a man trailing me in an old truck.

He left enough distance to keep from arousing my suspicions, I suppose. But every time I turned, he turned. I skirted the park but drove normally—right to the nearest police station.

When I pulled into the parking lot, he stopped under a shade tree across the street. I got a perfect description of his truck for the police before he pulled away.

Consumer Tips: Keep Your Head or Lose Your Shirt

1. Hearing Aid Fraud—Check claims.
2. Death Vultures—Deal with reputable funeral home.
3. Health Quackery—Select reputable doctors.
4. Real Estate Schemes—Take time to investigate.
5. Home Repair Rackets—Check with Better Business Bureau.
6. Work-at-Home Schemes—Check with BBB.
7. Medigap Insurance Double-Policy Schemes—Choose a reliable agent.
8. Bank Examiner Scam—Call police.
9. "Pack Game" (finding money)—Call police.

Keeping alert to the above list of popular scams and what to do to avoid becoming a victim should spare you money and trouble. But not all those out to get you are dressed as wolves. Some wear sheep's clothing. For example:

When I answered the phone the other night, the caller identified himself and his organization and said he was taking orders for American flags. "Proceeds from the sale of these flags," he said, "go to buy wheelchairs for veterans."

What a worthy cause for only a $14.95 investment!

Suddenly I remembered a consumer report. The reporter learned that the local VA hospital had plenty of wheelchairs; the fund raising was only a gimmick.

Before hanging up, I told the caller I had heard about his organization. I hope he got the message.

Whether you're in a high, middle, or low income bracket, you can bet your bottom dollar that before you go to sleep tonight, someone will try to get some of your money. Not a robber or burglar. Not necessarily a fraud. In all probability, legitimate operators will accost you. Not on the street or in a dark, dangerous alley. But right in your own home via your television, front door, mailbox, or telephone. Learning to resist these schemers will increase your chances of keeping what money you have to spend for what you want.

Probably the sneakiest culprit is TV. In spite of an innate resentment toward TV commercials, most viewers get the message. To keep your money requires that you scrutinize those TV commercials for flaws in logic—better yet, tune them out.

You know very well that Brand X toothpaste can't be the best, because a charming young actress with a perfect set of glistening teeth said on another channel a few seconds ago that she always uses Brand Y. The truth is, whatever brand you're using is probably as good as, and cheaper than, the touted brands. After all, someone has to pay advertising costs. Who else but the gullible viewer?

Why not try an experiment? Next time you're lonely or bored—otherwise why waste time on TV commercials?—and the models tell you that to be popular and happy, all you need is their soap, shampoo, deodorant, perfume, or breath freshener, turn off the TV. Take a shower with the soap you have, use your favorite shampoo, deodorant, perfume, and gum. Then take a friend or two out to dinner on part of the money you saved.

You're winning victory over TV commercials; you're actually saving money. Then, while you're congratulating yourself, a gorgeous blonde appears on the screen driving or caressing the sleek latest model of your four-year-old car. If you buy the car this week, you'll get a one-thousand dollar rebate. WOW!

Before reaching for your checkbook, think. Did the ad quote a price? What about the trade-in value of your car? Is the dealer reliable? Do you really need a new car? Had you planned to buy a new car in the near future? What effect will buying a new car this week have on your budget? By letting someone else buy the "bargain," you pocket your share of the exorbitant advertising cost. And, more important, you're still in control of your own money.

Keep a mental list of items you need and organizations you want to support. Be wary of opening the door to any salesman or solicitor not represented on that list. Deal gently, but firmly, with such uninvited strangers. With their sales psychology, once inside your house, they will very likely leave with money you had no intention of spending. And leave you holding a product you hadn't the slightest intention of buying.

Her neighbors became suspicious when a widow with adequate income couldn't afford basic necessities. Investigation revealed that unscrupulous salesmen had sold her far more insurance than she needed, much of it duplicate coverage. The courts intervened in her case and forced the companies to refund her premiums for the excess insurance.

Two of my high school seniors invited my husband and

me to a "free" dinner. To avoid hurting the girls' feelings, we accepted their invitation. Had we given each a two-hundred-dollar graduation gift, we would have saved money. After a lovely meal, the genial hosts explained their company plans to make money for investors in their insurance stock. We had made some money in a similar venture. It sounded like a solid investment. Foolishly, we filled out a card, giving these "hosts" our name, address, and a convenient time for them to call on us.

They came to our house to discuss their plan further and to get our signature and check. We lost every dime we invested; friends whom we recommended lost their money, too. After unsuccessful attempts to locate the company office, I happened to notice a short newspaper item years later and learned that one of the chiselers had been sentenced to the State Penitentiary for taking money under false pretenses. Small consolation for the money we lost and the embarrassment over our friends' loss of money!

Maybe you have no trouble resisting the door-to-door salesman or even those who come at your invitation. But what about one who gains entrance into your home as a friend, an acquaintance, or even a serviceman?

Some time ago I called a serviceman. He was also a friend. Before leaving, he said, "I have something in the car I want to show you."

He dashed to the car and came back carrying a little box and some literature. Heading straight for the kitchen sink, he attached a water filter to the faucet. Then handing me the literature, he proceeded to tell us about the dangers of drinking city water and about the virtues of his special water filter.

In addition to the health factor, selling these water filters was providing him and other dealers with a "get-rich-quick" scheme. "You don't have to sell the filter; it sells itself. All you have to do is enlist other dealers, who in turn enlist others." The popular pyramid approach is used successfully to sell various products.

I said, "But somebody has to buy the product."

"Of course," he admitted, "every dealer has to buy one."
We told him we were not interested. But he left the filter. After he left, I read his literature. One book, obviously, the sales clincher, links chlorinated water with heart disease. It goes so far as to state that atherosclerosis cannot occur in the absence of chlorinated water.

Almost instantly I recalled at least four members of my family who died with a stroke or heart attack; none of whom had lived in a city or drunk chlorinated water. Down the drain went that argument.

Keep a huge wastebasket near the front door. Even the innocent postman comes every day, his mail bag bulging with schemes to get your money.

If you don't contribute to your political party, the results will be disastrous. If you don't contribute to a certain radio or TV evangelist, he will be forced to go off the air, he says in his letter. Tough luck! If you will present a certificate at the office of a certain recreational resort developer, you will receive luxurious accommodations while you view the development and subject yourself to high-pressure sales tactics.

Or if you will call a certain number or appear at a certain place within a specified period of time, you will definitely get a prize, ranging from a Polaroid camera to a new Cadillac. If you don't send in those Sweepstakes Certificates, you deserve to spend the rest of your life in poverty. Occasionally someone does win, of course, but your chances are virtually nil. All these offers sound tempting, however, because they are professionally designed.

The most ridiculous scheme I ever saw was a letter from a man in Arizona. Attributing his "secret formula" to "the Man upstairs," the writer outlined how much money various numbers of people would need to send him to make him a millionaire—a dream he had always had. He decided to settle for what seemed to him the most logical way to reach his goal: to send 1,000 letters to 1,000 people, asking for a lifetime non-interest loan of $1,000 per person. He promised to "invest in secure, long-term obligations, which will provide a constant (year after year) flow of income. Then live a quiet, peaceful remaining few years, doing little things for other people—just like you have done for me." Little things?

After disregarding TV commercials, banishing the persistent salesman, and tossing your scheme letters into the trash, you still have another, more urgent, more persistent, nuisance to deal with, your telephone.

You're stuck with Bell's invention. You dare not throw it out. How can you deal with undesirable telephone solicitations? Here are a few suggestions you might try:

First, establish a policy never to buy anything from anyone who calls you on the phone. Any business that has to resort to such tactics probably isn't doing much anyhow, maybe because it isn't reliable. For every dollar you lose by not taking advantage of those enticing telephone offers, you'll probably save ten. The "don't call me, I'll call you" philosophy would be a good business motto.

Second, interrupt the caller's memorized sales pitch to ask questions. For example, when a lady called me recently to inform me that my husband and I had been selected to receive two cemetery lots "free," she asked when we would be at home so a company representative could deliver the deeds. I asked, "What's the catch?" No catch, she assured me. All we had to do was to listen for thirty minutes to their salesman explain their "plan." She hinted that we had friends, of course, who would be interested in buying cemetery lots. I said, "No, thanks," and hung up. We still don't have cemetery lots, but we'll probably buy them when we're ready, with no strings attached.

Third, I realize many of you will be shocked at my next suggestion, but the phone belongs to you; hang up when you please. Nothing convinces a caller that you mean "No" quicker than the click of the receiver followed by a dial tone. Rude? Sure. What do you call interrupting whatever you're doing—often eating or sleeping—to tell you something you don't want to hear and try to get money you don't want to spend? Presumptuous, as well as rude.

When our friend Mr. Davis answered the telephone one morning, a man identifying himself as a bank official asked for help in catching a teller suspected of embezzlement. Mr. Davis could help, the caller said, by going to the bank and withdrawing his savings from this teller's window. By practicing this deception on others less alert, the crook had perfected a plausible story.

When the man hung up, however, Mr. Davis called his bank. Bank officials advised him to cooperate in the scheme. Police caught the racketeer when he came to check on Mr. Davis' money.

Most of us know how we want to spend our money. We have a budget. We plan our purchases. But unless we learn to say "No" to high-pressure sales pitches, we may not be able to spend our money as we want to. Be a tough customer, if you must. It's your money. The sale doesn't have to begin when the prospective customer says, "No." It can end there.

If something sounds too good to be true, it probably is. If you keep your cool, you can keep your cash.

Now that you know how to keep from losing your shirt, let's see how well you can apply that knowledge. I've designed a simple test to let you determine your response.

Just How Gullible Are You?

Unsuspecting people all around you are victimized every day by con artists. Your chances of becoming a victim depend largely on your gullibility. Your answers to the following questions should help you evaluate your level of susceptibility.

Situation I: You're approaching your car in the parking lot of a shopping mall. A stranger walks up to you and says: "I've just found $5,000." She shows you a paper bag. "I don't know what to do with it. I'm afraid I'll be accused of stealing it. I need help. I can't afford to risk getting caught with this money. I've got to see my lawyer and find

out what to do. If you'll take me to my lawyer's office, I'll give you $200."
Would you
A.___ Take her
B.___ Get in the car and leave her standing there
C.___ Dash into a store and call the police
D.___ Other: _____

Situation II: You have just cashed a check at your bank. As you walk away, a foreigner steps up and says, in broken English: "I have just inherited $10,000 from my uncle. I can't take it back to my country with me; they'll think I stole it. I want to give it to the Salvation Army. If you will take me there, I'll give you $250.
Would you
A.___ Take him to the Salvation Army
B.___ Give him the brush off
C.___ Go back inside the bank and call police
D.___ Other: _____

Situation III: Your purse or wallet is stolen from the restroom in a department store. After reporting the loss, you rush home. The telephone rings. A voice says: "This is Anita Long from the department store. Your purse (or wallet) has been found. You can pick it up at the credit desk."
Would you
A.___ Hurry to the store
B.___ Notify the police
C.___ Ask a friend to pick it up
D.___ Other: _____

Situation IV: A truck turns into your driveway. A man comes to the door and says: "We're resurfacing driveways in this area, and we just happen to have a little tar left over. I noticed your driveway needs some tar. We'll make you a special price just to get rid of what we have left." He quotes a bargain price, maybe $75.00.

Would you
A. __ Accept his offer
B. __ Reject his offer
C. __ Check with the Better Business Bureau
D. __ Other: _____

Situation V: Two women get out of a car and come to your door. "We're from the telephone company," they tell you. "We'd like to inspect your phone."
Would you
A. __ Invite them in
B. __ Call the telephone company's business office
C. __ Call the police
D. __ Other: _____

Situation VI: You get a notice in the mailbox. It says: "We've been trying to deliver a package. Please call 950-6814 to arrange for delivery."
Would you
A. __ Dial that number
B. __ Call the Better Business Bureau
C. __ Throw the notice away
D. __ Other: _____

Situation VII: A woman rings your doorbell. When you open the door, she says: "I've got a flat. Could I use your phone to call my husband?"
Would you
A. __ Let her in
B. __ Offer to call for her
C. __ Slam the door in her face
D. __ Other: _____

Situation VIII: A friend's daughter invites you to a dinner an out-of-town company is hosting for high school seniors in your city.
Would you
A. __ Think of an excuse to refuse the invitation

25

B.___Check with the Better Business Bureau
C.___Blindly accept the invitation
D.___Other:_____

Situation IX: In the mail you receive a notice that you have won a 25″ color television set. All you have to do is call the office for an appointment to pick it up.
Would you
A.___Disregard the notice
B.___Call the office immediately
C.___Check with the Better Business Bureau
D.___Other:_____

Situation X: Your telephone rings. The caller says: "This is John Smith. I'm on the board of First National Bank. We suspect one of our tellers of embezzling money. But we need your help to catch her. I'm sure that, as a good citizen, you are willing to do your part to catch a criminal. We need you to go to her window and draw out your savings."
Would you
A.___Slam the receiver down
B.___Hang up politely and call your bank
C.___Cooperate
D.___Other:_____

Hopefully, answering the questions has made you think of options. Option D was included to encourage you to consider others not listed. Whatever your response, if this test tends to make you less gullible, it has accomplished its purpose.

No one can give you a pat answer for every possible situation. But reviewing methods by which some have handled these crises may point us in the right direction.

Situation I: Mrs. B., a middle-aged lady, agreed to take the stranger to the lawyer's office. She waited in the car until the stranger came out. Explaining that the lawyer's fee was $250, the "finder of $5,000" asked to borrow that amount. Mrs. B. even went home to get $250 for her "friend," then saw the stranger disappear into the office building with Mrs. B.'s $250.

Situation II: Mr. Young went to the bank during his lunch hour to cash a check. Turning from the window with $110 in his hand, he met the foreigner who claimed to have inherited $10,000 that he wanted to give to the Salvation Army. A second foreigner joined them. The two talked Young into adding his $110 to the $10,000 offering. Young and the second foreigner were to split the money and each give it to the Salvation Army. In the exchange, Young discovered the foreigners had disappeared with his $110.

Situation III: The victim in this case rushed back to the store to retrieve her purse. When she left home, the person who stole her purse from the hanger on the door inside the restroom booth entered and burglarized her home.

Situation IV: The old "just-happened-to-have-some-leftover" scam still surfaces from time to time in various areas. The fleeced victim complains that the swindlers merely mess up the driveway. The job invariably costs double the estimate. And, after checking with local companies, the victim learns that he paid far more than a local contractor would have charged.

Situation V: Despite warnings by utility companies, the old ploy to gain entrance into a house by posing as company representatives continues to thrive. Employees drive trucks with the company emblems clearly displayed. Not only do those employees wear uniforms, but they wear badges as well. You can even call the business office if you aren't sure.

Situation VI: If you are gullible enough to check into the package-delivery scam, you'll likely have to pay dearly for the package. You later find some cheap item, worth a fraction of what you paid. Throwing the notice away will save you money.

A cruel variation of this scam includes delivering to your house a package for your neighbor. Of course, you wouldn't hesitate to pay any amount due. Alas, when the

27

neighbor returns, you learn that he or she didn't order the package.

Situation VII: This ploy—often tried on single women or the elderly—enables a con artist to get inside your home and gain your confidence. When her "husband" arrives, you're stuck with both of them in the house. An offer to call for someone eliminates the threat of admitting strangers into your home.

Situation VIII: When someone invites you to a "free" dinner sponsored by some unfamiliar company, you can bet your house and lot that will be the most expensive dinner you ever ate. That is, if you're gullible.

Situation IX: Victims of this trick—which, incidentally, comes in various guises—discover when they go to pick up their "prize" they must pay exorbitant fees, far more than the cheap item is worth. Unscrupulous dealers get rich on such schemes. Throwing the notice in the trash makes sense—and dollars too.

Situation X: Posing as police officers, two men asked a senior citizen for help in an embezzlement investigation. They went to the bank with the victim. After withdrawing $10,000 from his savings, the elderly man gave the money to the crooks. They promised to deposit it at a bank to see if it would be put into an account or embezzled. The rascals were later arrested.

Who knows? You may be the next target. But you don't have to be the next victim.

Auto Accident Prevention

Car Safety

1. Buckle up. Wearing seat belts may reduce your risk of serious injury or death by more than 50%.
2. When you park your car, (a) make sure to put it in "Park," (b) set the parking brake carefully, and (c) shut off the ignition.
3. As your eyesight begins to fail, be extremely cau-

tious. Quit driving if you can't see clearly.
4. If your reaction time becomes seriously impaired, stop driving.
5. Avoid driving at night or in bad weather, if you can.
6. Check brakes, lights, and tires periodically.
7. As a rule of thumb, drive in the right lane except when passing another vehicle.
8. Be courteous. It may save your life.
9. Keep alert.
10. Review your state operator's manual at least every time you renew your driver's license.

Had I ignored the first rule of auto safety, I wouldn't be here to tell you about the flying mattress.

In more than forty years of driving, I have visualized almost every conceivable road hazard a driver could possibly encounter. When I read or hear about a fatal accident, freak or otherwise, I try to imagine myself in that situation. Often I can think of a possible way out of such a crisis, if the driver were alert, constantly on the lookout for trouble. But never, in my wildest imagination, did I dream of seeing, much less confronting an airborne mattress. When I faced that ordeal, only a miracle and my seat belt, not my driving skill, prevented another fatality.

A strong wind was blowing that September afternoon as I drove east on I-40 toward Oklahoma City. Because of our state fair and rush-hour traffic, I chose to drive our Buick LeSabre instead of our economy car.

Approaching an exit on the right and a merging to two lanes from the left, I overtook two slow-moving trucks in the right lane.

Checking my rearview mirror and my speedometer—60 MPH—I signaled, pressed the accelerator, and pulled into the left lane.

At that moment, the wind lifted a new mattress from a west-bound pickup. Sailing across the wide median, the mattress literally appeared out of the air, landing diagonally, grazing the grill of my car.

Instantly I hit the brakes full force. Too late.

My car bounced, jerked toward the right, and flew toward the embankment past the exit ramp. My seat belt held me in place. When the car struck pavement again, I wrestled the steering wheel to keep from going over the steep bank. I finally stopped the car between the right lane and the exit ramp, facing west.

In front of me, past the ramp, the battered mattress bounced off the road and landed on a bank. I could see the holes my car made when it hit.

I didn't see the trucks again. At least they had cleared the right lane before I flew across it.

As traffic began to move normally again, I escaped down the exit ramp.

At the bottom of the ramp, a man stopped and came back to my car.

"Are you all right?" he asked.

"Yes, I'm o.k.," I assured him. "Let's see if my car's all right."

"You nearly scared me to death," he said. "Your car completely left the pavement."

We decided the car wasn't damaged.

Later that evening, I noticed a slight scratch on my right leg. And when I took the car to the garage a few days later, the wheels were out of alignment. A far cry from a fatality or even a serious accident that only a miracle and a seat belt could have prevented. Turning a big car like that around in two and one-half lanes—at 60 plus miles per hour? Impossible! Yet true.

Speaking of turning, it's time to move on.

Chapter 4
Bella Vista Boulevard: Behavioral Sciences Center

We're turning right onto Bella Vista Boulevard. Our first stop here will be the social service center. We'll gain information on how to deal with the identity crisis, how to build self-esteem, and how to adapt to our changing life style.

From there, we'll move on to the Community College, where we'll learn to respect and enrich our intellectual capacities. We'll meet other senior citizens involved in adult educational opportunities.

A brief life review should prepare us for this area of our tour.

Shakespeare describes seven ages of man: (1) the infant, (2) the schoolboy, (3) the lover, (4) the soldier, (5) the justice, (6) Pantaloon, (7) second childishness.[1] We laugh with the poet until we recognize in the mirror a close resemblance to Pantaloon—the clown.

"That can't be me," we insist. "Who is this?" we ask.

Unmistaken Identity

Retirement inevitably forces us into a new role. Most of us adjust to the transition with comparative ease. We've rather looked forward to the various stages, at least thus far. For some, however, the crisis proves traumatic.

"Who am I?" we may ask.

A satisfactory answer lays a foundation for our acceptance of our new role.

In his essay "Who Precisely Do You Think You Are?" Archibald MacLeish asks a crucial question. Coping successfully with all crises depends upon our response.

Moses was eighty years old when God spoke to him from

31

a burning bush. After grooming this potential leader from his infancy, God was ready to use him.

"You're to go before Pharaoh and persuade him to release the Children of Israel," God explained. "Then you're to lead the Israelis to the land I promised to give them."

Suddenly Moses got cold feet—and taking off his shoes had nothing to do with it. One translator records his reaction:

"But Moses said to God, 'I'm a nobody. How can I go to the king and bring the Israelites out of Egypt?'" (Ex. 3:11).

Imagine that! Brought up as a prince in Pharaoh's house, trained in the decorum surrounding royalty, he, of all Hebrews, should know how to approach a king. No doubt God let the princess find the infant Moses in the water for the very purpose of preparing him for this task. Obviously God didn't consider him a "nobody."

One of my favorite mottoes declares: "God didn't make no junk."

In *The Death of a Salesman*, Willy Loman commits suicide at the end of a phony existence. His son Biff says of him "He never knew who he was." He always pretended to be someone he wasn't—a decent husband and father, a successful business man, a big shot.

How sad!

Our very sanity may depend on our answer to the identity question. In *Search for Identity*, Earl Jabay tells of touring a mental hospital with a chaplain.

Explaining the illnesses of various patients, the minister said, "The basic question which these people are asking is . . . 'Who am I?'" He went on to say that one patient thought he was Christ; another claimed to be Napoleon; a third said he was an animal.[2]

To arrive at a logical conclusion as to who you are, we might first consider who or what you are not.

When a stranger asks, "Who are you?" you tell him your name. If your name is John Brown, for example, it certainly doesn't identify you, nor any of the other John Browns listed on page after page of telephone books. You wouldn't want to be mistaken for one of them. Like my husband, you might hear your name on a news bulletin reporting the surrender of a plane hijacker. If you're a woman, you may change your name when you marry, but your identity doesn't change. The "rose by any other name would smell as sweet." Your name is not unique; you are.

You are not a relationship. Although some relish living in the shadow of their spouse, you would probably resent being introduced as "Dr. Prominent Citizen's wife" or "Mrs. Vice-President's husband." You may cringe when introduced as "Dr. Famous Person's son." "You'll never be the preacher your father is"—the statement from the lips of a prominent man humiliated a young minister whose father was a great orator. No matter how many outstanding people are on your family tree, you are not your family. It's gratifying to remember that statement when you know of infamous family members too.

In this age of high technology, it would be easy to consider yourself just a machine or a number. But you are not even a wheel or a cog in a wheel. You are not a social security number nor a credit card number, not even a telephone or house number or zip code.

You are not a color—red, black, or white. Nor are you a problem—cancer patient, schizophrenic, or failure.

You are not an animal. Columnist Ferdie J. Deering attacks the tendency of many scientists to accept and teach theory for fact. He says, "Too many scientists or pseudoscientists seem to have no partitions in their brains to separate facts and imagination."[3]

No scientific hypothesis has been more touted as fact than the theory that man evolved from an animal. But this theory raises more questions than it answers.

This idea may strike you as surprising, but you are not a title, profession, or job. You may have various titles within your profession. You may change professions. You may lose your job. You may retire. But your identity remains constant. You are not what you do.

You are not a mere human body. Several years ago

someone analyzed the chemical elements in an average-sized man. He broke down the ingredients as follows:
>   Enough fat to make seven bars of soap,
>   Enough iron to make a 10-penny nail,
>   Enough sulphur to rid a small dog of fleas,
>   Enough phosphorus to put the heads on a book of matches,
>   Enough starch for a small family laundry,
>   Enough sugar to fill a large sugar bowl,
>   And a few miscellaneous elements.

The total value was $1.98 at that time—probably $12 or $13 now.

But intuition assures you that you are of infinite value. You are far more than a body.

You are not a robot. Sigmund Freud taught that our choices are foreordained by hidden psychic forces. Whatever we feel, say, or do is the product of the instinctual forces in the unconscious mind, he claimed. If this be true, we can evade all responsibility. Our behavior may be "unhealthy," but not "evil."

*MacLeish warns that a person may "miss his life if he doesn't know who's living it—if he thinks a lawyer is living it or a professor of biochemistry or the head of a dry-cleaning plant or a mechanical engineer." For example, a man suddenly wakes up in middle age only to find that instead of him in his bed, it's an officer of the bank. Worse yet, a woman may "come to herself . . . only to discover that she has no self to come to." Instead, there's only "the children's nurse or the chauffeur of the family station wagon, or the fourth chair in a bridge game."[4]

Since you may miss your life if you don't know who's living it, the identity question is vital. Fortunately, the Bible provides a simple answer: You are a soul, created in the "image of God." "And the LORD God formed man *of*

---

* From "Who Precisely Do You Think You Are?" in A CONTINUING JOURNEY by Archibald MacLeish. Reprinted by permission of Houghton Mifflin Company.

the dust of the ground, and breathed into his nostrils the breath of life; and man became a living soul" (Gen. 2:7). You don't just *have* a soul; you *are* a soul.

The Patriarch Job asked God: "What *is* man, that thou shouldest magnify him?" (Job 7:17). David, the psalmist, elaborates:

> What is man, that thou art mindful of him? and the son of man, that thou visitest him?
>
> For thou hast made him a little lower than the angels, and hast crowned him with glory and honour.
>
> Thou madest him to have dominion over the works of thy hands: thou hast put all *things* under his feet:
>
> All sheep and oxen, yea, and the beasts of the field;
>
> The fowl of the air, and the fish of the sea, *and whatsoever* passeth through the paths of the seas (Psalm 8:4-8).

Through Hamlet, Shakespeare says of this noble creature:

> What a piece of work is man! how noble in reason! how infinite in faculties! in form and moving how express and admirable! in action how like an angel! in apprehension how like a God! the beauty of the world, the paragon of animals![5]

Lifting man to his loftiest pinnacle, Jesus taught him to address God as "Our Father." How could anyone say, "I'm a nobody"? When I was a child, I used to hear Christians testify that they were weak worms of the dust. What an insult to God! We're His children.

Saint Paul speaks of the Christian as a part of the Body of Christ and the Bride of Christ.

How exciting to know that God loves us so much! We are so special that Jesus said the very hairs of our head are numbered.

Failing to learn one's identity leads to insecurity and

emotional turmoil. But finding out "precisely" who he is enables one "not to think *of himself* more highly than he ought to think; but to think soberly, according as God hath dealt to every man the measure of faith" (Rom.12:3).

"No small part of the problems of those who receive treatment for emotional problems is that they have lost their sense of identity,"6 Jabay declares. If that statement is true, finding our identity is crucial to mental health.

According to an old fable, when God created man and the animals, He gave to each a life span of twenty years. The horse, the deer, the dog, the monkey, for example—each had twenty years.

The horse called a meeting of all the animals. In recognition of his common sense, the other animals made the horse chairanimal of the convention. Few realized the significance of the traumatic decisions the Chair hoped to generate during the business session.

"It's a shame," the Chair began, "that man, who is so much more intelligent than we are, has only twenty years to live."

"If it's agreeable to the rest of you, I'll give man ten years of my life," he added.

Several other animals went along with the plan. The deer, the dog, and the monkey each gave man ten years.

The moral of the story is this: The first twenty years of a man's life, he really lives. The next ten years, he works like a horse. The next ten, he runs like a deer. The next ten, he leads a dog's life. From then on, he just monkeys around.

At any rate, we're familiar with role changes. Since we've weathered the forties, however, we should be able to adjust to almost anything.

Coming to terms with the identity question enables us to avoid the greatest problem in accepting the retirement role—poor self-image, uselessness, isolation, and aimlessness. Without a good self-image, the loss of job role—"I used to be a ____ ," "Now I am a ____ "—can be quite devastating, especially for a woman who faces divorce or widowhood.

Moving successfully from a job to the retirement role, however, demands more than a good self-concept. It requires financial and physical independence and the ability to make decisions—self-determination.

The retirement role includes the right to financial support without working full time, to management of time and other resources, and to all privileges afforded other citizens.

In return, the retiree feels certain obligations to society to share expertise with others; to volunteer services occasionally; to avoid full-time employment; to accept responsibility for decision-making concerning his own life; and to avoid, as long as possible—becoming dependent.

Psychologist Robert Peck believes that what an old person loses in "physical stamina, strength, and attractiveness," he must compensate for in "wisdom or mental energies." He must use past experience to solve everyday problems. Failure to replace physical loss with mental achievements results in bitterness and disillusionment.[7]

With children leaving home, the death of family members and friends, and retirement, the older person must make new contacts and seek new activities or become depressed. To adapt, he must have a flexible, not a rigid, mind.

Anxiety and depression are not automatic. But often healthy retirees complain of headaches, gastrointestinal problems, irritability, nervousness, and lethargy.

These symptoms of the "retirement syndrome" are increased by confusion of roles, activities, and changes in life structure. Without a satisfying life style and work supplements, these symptoms worsen. "A sense of inadequacy can evolve; and apathy and inertia and what some have called 'senile' behavior may follow unless the condition is prevented or reversed."[8]

Negative Emotions

At times even the most positive thinker battles negative

emotions. An acquaintance of a possibility thinking advocate said of him: "I've seen him on the bottom rung of the ladder."

No matter how healthy our mental attitudes, sometimes situations beyond our control shatter our dreams and leave us devastated—at least temporarily. Aging often makes us especially vulnerable to low moods.

Boredom

Most retirees relish a few weeks or even months of relief from punching the clock. We enjoy freedom to do as we please. We like release from a rigid schedule.

But once we catch up with what we planned before retirement, we may tire of so much leisure. Some of us long for a fixed schedule. If we aren't disciplined, we tend to give up and die in our shell. We sometimes bore others because we depend on them to entertain us.

Loneliness

On the heels of boredom comes loneliness. If living, our spouse may still be working or involved in his or her own interests. Our children have little time to spare. Friends aren't so entertaining as they were at first. Often family members and friends move away or die.

We live more and more in the past. We need opportunities to reminisce, to go back to our roots. But we notice that most people aren't interested in listening. Unless we cultivate friends among our age group, we may feel like the lady who said, "There's no place in today's society for old people and children. You have to get in, get out, or get run over."

Everyone knows what it's like to be lonely. Probably no one has escaped its depressing presence completely. Few sights provoke our pity more than that of an elderly person in the throes of loneliness. Sitting alone day after day with little opportunity to talk to anyone saps the zest for living. Especially sad is the parent who wastes away in a nursing home, forsaken by busy children and uncaring grandchildren.

But if loneliness gives way to self-pity, the victim drives away the very cure for his or her negative emotion.

Most people believe the elderly are the loneliest group in our society. Surveys, however, indicate the opposite. According to Dr. Joyce Brothers, "Surveys indicate adolescents are the loneliest group in our society."[9]

One reason for our isolation is that "most of us go through life wearing a series of masks," Doctor Brothers says. She blames much of our loneliness on the fact that "we are very clever at hiding our real selves," so clever, in fact, that some of us "don't even know who we are."[10]

Marriage is not a cure for loneliness, Doctor Brothers insists, for being alone and being lonely are not the same thing. But when we're alone, it's more difficult "to evade ourselves."[11]

To cope with loneliness, she offers several suggestions:
1. Accept the blame. Stop blaming others.
2. Make the effort to get out and meet people.
3. Join political organizations or other groups.
4. Saunter through parks, zoos, art galleries, or museums. Talk to people. Ask questions.
5. Join in sports activities where you meet poeple.[12]

Frustration

We're used to having a salary to depend on. Usually we could expect a raise periodically. We've always felt like getting up in the morning and doing whatever we wanted to do. We've enjoyed our family, our friends, and our work. We've made plans and carried them out.

Now we're on a fixed income. Sometimes we don't feel like getting up and doing what we want or need to do. We're losing family members, friends, and maybe even our mate. We still make plans, but carrying them out sometimes poses problems. We're forced to admit, "I can't do what I once could." With so many limitations, naturally we feel frustrated.

Tension

For years we've called the shots in our home if not at work. After retirement we may discover that people talk down to us. We sense that the value of our opinion has greatly diminished. We are expected to subject our will to that of others. We find it hard to relinquish our place of authority. Yet we fight against resentment and bitterness. Sometimes the tension drives us to the breaking point.

Depression

If we allow our minds to feed on these negative emotions, we're likely to join the ranks of the depressed.

Pity Me: I'm Depressed

I don't want to get up;
I don't want to get dressed.
I prefer to do nothing;
Just call me depressed.

I don't care how I look;
I don't comb my hair;
I've put on some weight
And don't care what I wear.

I lock doors and windows
And pull down the blinds;
I just can't face people
Who have carefree minds.

I scream at my children;
I yell at my mate,
Blame them and my parents
For my miserable fate.

I muster a headache
When my mate desires sex;
And I couldn't care less
If our marriage it wrecks.

Don't tell me to shape up;
I'll continue to mope;
I've had such a hard life
That I simply can't cope.

I've consulted five doctors
But each of them said,
There's nothing the matter;
It's all in my head.

I've gone to a counselor
With my tale of woes;
But straight down the drain
All that good money goes,

Along with his counsel,
Which I really don't heed,
Because deep in my heart
I know what I need.

I refuse to admit it
But the truth of it is,
I'm possessed with self-pity,
And I like it like this.
—Barkley

Admittedly, some people suffer physical and emotional problems that cause depression. For those victims, we all have the utmost sympathy. But others like the one pictured here need something besides pity.

Fear

Since even the most faithful—in this sense full of faith—sometimes succumb to fear, we might consider some methods of dealing with fear to determine the most effective means for us.

1. We can whine. "Why did this happen to *me?*" The answer is simple: "Because I'm human."

2. We can rebel. Often a "Why-n-ing" attitude leads to rebellion. "If God loved me, He wouldn't let me go through this." Rebellion increases fear and adds its own torture.

3. We can panic. This, of course, is no solution.

4. We can pray. The Psalmist David declares: "I sought the LORD, and he heard me, and delivered me from all my fears" (Ps. 34:4). Compared to David, most of us don't know what fear is.

5. After praying, we can trust. Evidently "Fear not" was one of Jesus' favorite expressions. "Let not your heart be troubled" (John 14:1), He said to His friends in their darkest hour. His promise "lo, I am with you alway" enabled those men to face whatever the established religion and the Roman Empire could throw at them. We can put our trust in a God like that.

Positive Attitudes

Self-Confidence

I heard a speaker try this experiment:

"Think of one thing you like about yourself," she said. "Then raise your hand."

After a period of silence, one or two hands rose slowly and timidly to half-mast.

More silence and waiting. Finally a few more hands

went up.

"Now, I want you to think of one thing you don't like about yourself," she continued. "Then raise your hand."

Without hesitation, hands shot up all over the room.

The speaker explained that she had tried that experiment with elementary students, teenagers, and adults. Always with the same result.

Why? Probably because false humility has become so deeply engrained in us that we automatically concentrate on what we don't like about ourselves. We tend to remember our failures more vividly than our successes.

Saint Paul has the answer to false humility. He declares: "I can do all things through Christ which strengtheneth me" (Phil. 4:13).

Enthusiasm

Dale Carnegie said: "Act enthusiastic and you'll be enthusiastic."

Lest we lose our enthusiasm for today and tomorrow, we must continue to pursue our dream.

As a young husband and father, my grandfather had a dream. He wanted to found a Christian college. He donated ten acres of his farm land. He arranged for a college administrator to move there and initiate construction. He enlisted the help of neighbors to form a board of regents. He helped draw up plans for the first building. He ordered some of the lumber and other building materials and stored them on the donated site.

He was convinced that God had helped him buy a farm with a marketable mineral on it for the express purpose of building that college. In spite of his meager income, he gave relentlessly of his strength and money to accomplish what he thought was God's will for him.

World War II escalated. Educational leaders of his denomination decided they didn't need any more colleges at that time. A local church burned.

The administrator and his family moved on. The board

decided to use the lumber and other materials to rebuild the church that had burned. Finally an initial small indebtedness forced the sale of the farm—including the ten donated acres. Despite all evidence to the contrary, Grandfather kept the faith in his dream. As he aged, the vision increased in size and intensity.

After sixty years of struggle to build the college, he suffered a stroke. Realizing the impossibility of Grandfather ever achieving his goal, a minister friend said, "God will reward him as though the college were a reality." Perhaps. But, if not, the vision itself and striving to accomplish the task he firmly believed God wanted him to do kept him active far beyond the age when most of us give up. He died at age 95. Pursuing his dream kept up his enthusiasm.

Action

If "an idle mind is the devil's workshop," surely idle hands are instigators of negative emotions. Activity, within reason, dispels most boredom, loneliness, frustration, tension, and fear.

I've heard so many people say, "Since I retired I'm busier than I ever was" or "I don't know how I ever found time to work" that I'm determined to stop short of such frenzied activity. When my schedule gets too full, I deliberately cancel something. I have no intention of becoming overly involved.

On the other hand, I want a reasonable amount of activity, at least enough to keep away from negative thinking.

My husband and I moved across the street from Mary McCoy* soon after her husband died. We soon noticed that about six o'clock almost every evening, Mary would back out of her drive and head down the street. About ten o'clock we would hear her car slowing down and see her turn into the drive. I usually watched through a window until her light came on in the house.

* Names have been changed to protect the identity.

She explained that when she felt lonely, she would go visit a friend who didn't drive. Other widows joined them for games they all enjoyed.

Fran Johnson lives alone since her retirement. But she keeps busy. She works in a nursing home writing the biographies of those who live there.

With skills and time of volunteers in such demand, we have no excuse for not remaining as active as we want to be.

Faith

The story is told of a socialite in New York City who became so famous for her banquets that guests gladly flew in from distant cities for such occasions.

At one of those dinners she served a sumptuous delicacy—mushrooms. Reveling in the compliments of her guests, she knew her party was a success.

As she said "Goodnight" to the last guest, the hostess noticed her cat dash in through the door.

Guests scattered across the country.

Making a beeline for the kitchen, the cat jumped up on the cabinet and helped itself to the mushrooms. Within a matter of minutes, it fell over dead.

The astonished hostess called her doctor.

"Get in touch with all your guests. Tell them to have their stomachs pumped immediately," the doctor ordered.

In airports around the country, guests were paged. At three o'clock that morning, hospital emergency rooms were swamped with patients demanding that their stomachs be pumped.

"How's your cat?" a neighbor asked later that morning.

"Oh, my cat died last night. How did you know?"

"I'm so sorry. As I came home last night, your cat ran out in front of my car. I couldn't stop."

Doesn't such a story sound familiar? About the only exercise some of us get is jumping to conclusions. That's the story of our lives.

Oh, for the faith of a child!

Caught between his parents in a custody battle, Billy sensed the frustration and anxiety of his mother. Kneeling beside her on the eve of his return from spending three months with his dad, the three year old said, "Mother, God's going to take care of me. He put it right here in my head." The little fellow touched his forehead.

With so many problems and so much turmoil around us, if ever we needed faith it's now.

Love

How strange that everybody talks about love, everybody needs love, and everybody craves love; yet so many are starving for it!

Despite the "love-ins" and the superficial claims of "I love you," we see far too little evidence of the kind of love the Bible and Shakespeare talk about.

Divorce shatters the family, where love makes its greatest claims. Headlines reveal in gory detail stories of child abuse, rape, robbery, murder—often within a family setting.

A grandmother who seldom locked her doors becomes a victim of a savage murder. At the funeral, her grandson is arrested and charged with the crime. A high school student spends the night with a friend, stops by home and shoots his mother and step-father. A parent slowly murders his child by frequent beatings.

Is love still alive? Definitely.

Love is an act of will. God commands us to love one another. He gives us His quality of love if we're willing to accept it. If we love others we will be loved.

Activities

Hobbies

Most of us have at least one hobby. During our working years, we probably had little time and energy to devote to it. Now that we've retired, we can discover in it a source of pleasure and sometimes profit.

Art
As time permitted, Bill indulged in painting on and off the job. He has painted a number of pictures. Some sold for a good price. He took commercial art courses. He decorates store windows for Christmas, paints murals, and designs business cards and letterheads. Since retirement, he has time to pursue his hobby for enjoyment and extra income.

After his retirement, Paul bought tools and built a shop where he could indulge his hobby—wood carving. He probably hasn't sold enough to pay for his investment. But he enjoys making things to give away.

Karen makes dolls. She sells a few. The chief purpose, however, is therapy. She likes to keep busy and to create pretty dolls.

Carl plays the violin in the church orchestra. He gladly devotes the time each week to practice for the Sunday morning service. He's a retired college professor, but playing the violin is a hobby.

Writing
Susan is a retired English professor. She has just completed a book she wrote on assignment. Grace writes articles for her church periodicals. Carol is absorbed in writing a novel for one of her two creative writing classes at the university. None of these ladies has time to get bored or lonesome.

Reading
For those of us who like to read, retirement brings the leisure to pursue that hobby. A librarian in a small city expressed surprise that Mr. Davis, a man in his 80's, used the library more than almost anyone else in town. He liked to keep up with what was going on in the world. Until his death, he was an interesting conversationalist.

Figuring our income tax this year, I discovered that we are spending more for books and periodicals every year. My husband and I like to read. And reading makes a satisfying and worthwhile hobby.

Recreation

Everywhere we go we see senior citizens galore. We walk in the mall to avoid a heart attack. We play golf or tennis to keep in shape. We eat out because we don't like to cook, because the food tastes better, and because we can afford to. In the evening we watch TV, put together a puzzle, play Scrabble, or attend a concert.

Nowhere is the saying "once a man, twice a child" more evident than in the area of recreation. At last we have time for it, and we think we've earned it. And it helps prevent mental deterioration.

Travel

Whether you're on a tour, a cruise, or a camping trip, you'll meet hordes of Golden Agers. Many have dreamed of such excursions through months and years of punching the clock. Short vacations merely whetted our appetites for travel and adventure. No longer do we have to go back to work to rest from a vacation. If we come home tired, we can rest at home.

Travel agents and RV dealers thrive on this urge of senior citizens to travel while money and health hold out. A motto on some motor homes states: "We're living on the kid's inheritance." "Live it up" is the rule.

Social Activities

Most of us decide how active we want to be socially. In some churches senior citizens meet several times a week. For a token fee, they can eat lunch or they can take a dish as a contribution. They play games or do handcrafts with peers.

Our church sponsors a dinner once a month for senior adults. We take a dish and contribute a dollar to pay for the meat. We usually have a speaker to address issues important to our age group. We enjoy the food and the fellowship, as we gain information.

Sunday School classes plan social events each month. Sometimes we have a dinner, sometimes refreshments, sometimes games, sometimes a speaker or musical entertainment. Occasionally we furnish our own music.

Small groups of friends often get together to play games in homes or to eat out. Single retirees spend additional time together.

Garden clubs, bowling leagues, and golf games provide entertainment for the socially inclined.

If we aren't careful we tend to become overly involved.

Volunteer Work

From a block walker for the American Cancer Society or the March of Dimes campaign to the grey lady or candy striper in your local hospital, volunteers make an invaluable contribution. Without block walkers, the cost of collecting would far outweigh the value of the donations. Without grey ladies and candy stripers, hospital costs would escalate even more.

Despite the high visibility of paid staff, with rare exceptions, volunteers do much of the church work. Ideally, paid staff equip and enable laymen to serve in a wide variety of positions. For every hired worker, a church needs scores of volunteers. The larger the membership, the greater the need. One church, for example, submitted to its congregation a list of 116 jobs and asked for volunteers to fill those positions.

Almost every non-profit organization needs more volunteers than it has.

In addition to monetary benefits for the organization, volunteer service offers a sense of accomplishment, a feeling of self-satisfaction, and an antidote to loneliness and boredom.

Part-time Employment

For various reasons a retiree often prefers to work part time. Social Security seldom covers living expenses. Even an additional retirement pension and possible savings may prove inadequate. Working part time may well be the only way to afford extras—a new car, new furniture, new clothes, recreation, home repairs, travel.

Those with adequate resources may work part time to avoid giving up, to use job skills, or to feel needed and wanted.

Whatever the motive, a retiree should have no problem finding a part-time job. A professional person can usually find opportunities to use his or her expertise. A blue collar worker can find a market for his or her skills. An unskilled laborer has a wide selection of part-time jobs available. Newspaper Want Ads, combined with word-of-mouth information, should provide adequate leads.

Hopefully, you can find part-time work that affords a sense of dignity and accomplishment in keeping with your pre-retirement life style.

Golden Acres Community College

We are now on the campus of Golden Acres Community College. Before beginning our tour of these facilities, you might be interested in what research proves about the intellectual capacity of senior adults.

A study by the National Institute of Mental Health, coordinated by Dr. James E. Birsen and later by Dr. Robert N. Butler, found "psychological flexibility, resourcefulness, and optimism" among older people.

Men over 65 had "brain physiological and intellectual functions that compared favorably with those of a young control group. Intellectual abilities did not decline as a result of specific diseases." They concluded: "Therefore 'senility' is not an inevitable outcome of aging."

Other studies, such as one at Duke University, showed similar results. "All the usual psychiatric disorders found among the elderly seemed to be similar in genesis and structure to those affecting the young."[13]

"Severe psychologic decline is not an inevitable part of the aging process."[14]

Dr. Robert N. Butler concludes: "We've come to realize that aging is not simply a downhill course. We do continue to grow and develop throughout life. Judgment, experience and creativity do further unfold with time."[15]

Dr. Werner K. Shaie, Penn State University, made a study of memory and reasoning in the elderly. He concludes: ". . . (M)any participants maintained their prowess well into their 70's, and . . . a number actually improved their scores, including some in the 75 to 80 age bracket."

Shaie believes that those who "consider mental decline a natural part of aging" may "ignore symptoms that really derive from treatable physical disease or from reversible depression."

"Forgetfulness," Shaie says, "is no longer considered a 'normal' part of aging." The fact that people can't remember recent events, he believes, is usually a physical problem.

Shaie thinks much so-called senility is Alzheimer's disease.[16]

Alex Comfort says, "In the absence of ill health, such as untreated high blood pressure, aging has no adverse effect on intelligence or learning power. . . ."[17]

Educational Opportunities

With so many older people and so few young people in comparison, institutions of higher education now offer incredible incentives for senior citizens to enroll. Considering counting heads a top priority, these institutions court the retiree with short courses in whatever interests him or her or with a degree program.

While teaching in a junior college, I had scores of these elderly students in my classes. Helen, a lady in her 80's, had taught in rural schools until her retirement. Since she was teaching somewhere when I was born, I always felt a bit embarrassed when she slipped up to the desk and asked, "May I be excused?" But she enjoyed the class and the activities the college sponsors for senior adults.

Lucille, another elderly student, graduated from the junior college with excellent grades.

After her three doctor sons and a teacher daughter had finished college, Jane enrolled in a university. A friend asked, "Why are you going to college? Do you plan to teach during the Millennium?" But she continued her 60-mile drive each way until she moved entirely too far away from the university.

Mollie worked on her doctorate until she was in her 60's. Her granddaughter said, "Grandmother, if you get that degree, it will look good in your obituary."

A number of colleges and universities permit senior citizens to enroll on a space-available basis without tuition and fees. Such an arrangement gives the older person undreamed of educational opportunities.

Second Career

With easy availability of educational opportunities, a retiree may choose a second career. If he or she decides to retire early, say fifty-five or sixty, the worker may still have ample time for a new career.

For a retiree who wants to remain active, time and resources for advancement and pleasure abound.

Butler defines good mental health in old age as "the capacity to thrive rather than simply survive."[18]

"Old people become crazy . . . because they were crazy when young, because they have an illness, or because we drive them crazy."[19]

Chapter 5
Blue Ridge Heights: Marriage and Family Arena

"Can love and romance really last?" Mary, a gorgeous blonde with stars in her eyes, asked me.

"My parents are divorced," she explained. "My husband's parents are breaking up. My friends at work just laugh at me when I get sentimental about my husband. They insist it won't last.

"It scares me," she continued, "because he and I love each other. We have a happy marriage. But we're afraid that will all change when we get older."

Despite the odds, however, love is a matter of will. If we continue to love a person, it's because we will to do so. Where there's a will, there's a way to keep a marriage from going on the rocks.

Counselors here on Blue Ridge Heights specialize in helping us adjust to changing relationships inherent in aging. They assure us that change is often for better, not for worse. It's largely up to us, however, to make it better.

Let's stop here and see what we can learn.

Changes in Relationships

A retiree experiences a sudden separation from the job, a probable decrease in income, and a loss of his former role. Along with these, he may face dramatic changes in intimate and not so intimate relationships. Adapting to these challenges requires infinite patience and a flexible mind.

Spouse

A former executive said to a friend: "You know, since I retired, I've gotten rid of my ulcer. But now my wife has one."

In many cases that statement may very well prove true. When both have gone to a job five days a week and come home—maybe bringing work from the office or doing household chores—the couple worked out a satisfactory routine. They had relatively little time to spend together at home.

Unless they plan specifically for time alone, as retirees they get under each other's feet. Especially does the wife wish her husband wasn't around all the time. She can't get as much done. And he mopes around like a restless child asking, "Mother, what can I *do?*"

A wife who has not worked outside the home may feel even more resentment toward a husband who invades "her" domain.

What may have been a cherished reason for retirement—togetherness—may well turn into a nightmare. To prevent such a catastrophe, each needs time and space to be alone. In addition to common objectives and interests, each needs personal goals and activities.

One couple who taught in the same school discovered they had so many common experiences that they had little to discuss at home in the evening. When the wife took another job, their communication took on greater interest. They had something to talk about.

Who knows? Maybe the old saying, "Familiarity breeds contempt" sprang from a retired couple who had allowed all their interests to converge. Variety keeps a marriage from growing stale.

Going everywhere together and doing everything together may suit some couples. For others, however, the changing relationship is less drastic if it allows room for privacy and individuality.

Sexuality

As a person ages, he or she often tends to change from viewing a mate as a sex object to that of a source of comfort and companionship. For some couples, however, sexual activity continues to play an important role in their relationship. They may trade quantity for quality. Nevertheless, they enjoy the intimacy they've had across the years.

Why not a sex revolution for senior citizens? Are we to let a sex-oriented society laugh us out of so much pleasure just because we're not so spry as we used to be?

We may lack the money to dress well, go to romantic settings, or even buy dentures and hearing aids. Yet we still crave the intimacy we've shared through the years. For most couples, even sexual intimacy can last a lifetime.

It is true that at least one study shows nearly 50% of the men are impotent by age 60.[1] But much impotence in older men is psychological. It can be overcome with counseling. If not psychological, it is treatable. Implants enable many men to function successfully after long periods of impotence.

Frequency of contact is not so important; each contact renews years of intimacy. "Each partner keeps the sense of being desirable and the identity of a sexually alive person."[2] "For many older people," says Isadore Rubin, "continued sexual relations are important not so much for the pleasurable release from sexual tension as for the highly important source of psychological reinforcement that they may provide.[3]

"Though the capacity for sexual response does slow down gradually, along with all the other physical capacities," continues Rubin, "it is usually not until actual senility that there is a marked loss of sexual capacity."[4] Rossman concludes: "There seems to be a growing and increasingly widespread belief that with appropriate therapy, all older people are going to have more capability in sexual performance."[5] How comforting to know that one of the strongest bonds holding a couple together through all the joys and sorrows of their married life will continue as a source of joy and strength, dispelling loneliness for both.

In spite of such encouragement, however, according to

Los Angeles psychologist, Paul Abramson, "To 90 percent of older people, menopause signalled the end of sexuality."[6] No doubt that situation accounts for the epidemic of twin beds or separate bedrooms for Grandpa and Grandma. "His snoring keeps me awake" or "I keep turning over and waking him up" may sound like a logical reason for separate beds. But at the very time we're depending more than ever on the closeness of a spouse, we move further apart at bedtime. We lack the warmth of our lover through the cold, dark hours of the night.

Masters and Johnson shed some light on our plight. They list five major factors limiting sexual response in women:
1. Steroid starvation, which makes coitus painful (estrogenic creams can often bring relief)
2. Lack of opportunity
3. Victorian concept that women shouldn't be interested
4. Physical infirmities of the partner
5. Never learning to respond—using menopause as an excuse for total abstinence

With proper therapy, there is no time limit on a woman's sexual capacity, especially if she remains sexually active throughout her adult life.

On the other hand, in men, performance wanes with age. "Yet for those older men who have established a high sexual output, by whatever means, in their middle years, there appears to be a much less significant decline." And, if health is maintained, they can maintain sexual output into the 80's.

Factors reducing the possibility of satisfactory sex are the following:
1. Boredom with partner
2. Preoccupation with career or economic pursuits
3. Mental or physical fatigue
4. Overindulgence in food or drink
5. Physical or mental infirmities
6. Fear of poor performance (very important, but women don't understand a man's fear of rejection)[7]

Poor health inhibits sex. Sometimes a woman fears she's no longer desirable and a man fears failure. So sex isn't resumed after the recovery of an ill mate.[8]

Probably the most prevalent of these fears is that of a couple after the man has suffered a heart attack. Recent studies, however, provide reassurance. "A number of studies have shown," says Isadore Rossman, "that the cardiac expenditure in intercourse is approximately that involved in climbing two flights of stairs."[9]

Doctors treating older people must deal with the following problems:
1. Absence of sexual desire
2. Self-punishment—guilt feelings
3. Boredom—lose sexual appetite—start skipping
4. Unrealistic expectations
5. Fear—myths
6. Physical problems—sometimes require adjustments
7. Degrees of male impotency
8. Degrees of female frigidity: lack of response, difficulty in achieving orgasm, lubrication
9. Bad advice, or no advice, from a family doctor (patients are reluctant to discuss and the doctor doesn't volunteer information)
10. Medications with a sexual side effect
11. Discrepancy in sexual desire and technique—poor communication[10]

Fortunately, almost all of these conditions can be treated and the problems resolved. But often we hesitate to mention such intimate concerns to a doctor. We're like the lady in the doctor's office. Her husband said, "Honey, tell the doctor where you hurt." "He ought to know," she snapped; "he's a doctor." Yes, but he waits for you to tell him your concerns. Then he can help.

Companionship

Jim was 94 when we took him to the nursing home to visit his 91-year-old wife. Jim walked straight to her room, shifted his cane to his left hand, and leaned over her bed.

"I finally got to come to see you," he said, his voice trembling.

"What?" Mary yelled back at him with a semiconscious stare.

"I said, 'I finally got to come to see you.' It's been over a week now since I've seen you. I thought the other day I was going to have to walk over here. I couldn't get anybody to bring me." His chin quivered.

"I don't know why I'm still here," Mary complained. "I'm no good to myself or anybody else anymore." She groaned as she turned to look at him.

"You're good for me," Jim assured her.

That scene and Jim's words impressed me primarily because my husband is Jim's son. I hope regardless of how ill or unattractive I may become in my final days, he will give me the assurance that I'm good for him.

Shakespeare expresses the thought in his lovely Sonnet 116:

Love's not Time's fool, though rosy lips and cheeks
Within his bending sickle's compass come;
Love alters not with his brief hours and weeks,
But bears it out even to the edge of doom.
If this be error and upon me proved,
I never writ, nor no man ever loved.[11]

One sure way to stifle romance is to neglect good personal hygiene and grooming. When you don't have to dress for the job, it's tempting to let yourself go.

Powder and perfume are no substitute for soap and water. Aunt Het, of the comics, said that when she tried to cover up her failure to bathe by using perfume, she felt like a hypocrite. She probably smelled like one, too.

At church one Sunday, I deliberately sat down beside an elderly widower who looked lonely. I had often seen him sitting alone. One whiff and I knew why. I found an excuse to move.

Tooth decay often causes bad breath without our knowledge.

A barber and a beautician are usually worth their cost, as aids to keeping romance alive, as well as building self-esteem.

And, ladies, for the sake of yourself and your husband and family, wear a dress often. Almost any man will tell you he likes his wife to wear a dress; she looks more feminine. He may not say so, but he doesn't want to look at you in a robe, jeans, or pant suit all the time. No, he may not say anything, but he may look at someone else.

Children

In her unique style, Erma Bombeck illustrates the normal role reversal between parent and child. Driving down the street one day, Erma had to stop suddenly. As she hit the brakes, she automatically reached her arm across to shield her mother. Erma realized their roles had changed. She had become the mother protecting the child.

Some time later, Erma was riding with her daughter. When the daughter made a sudden stop, she reached across to shield Erma. Their roles had reversed.

When children mature and leave home, a wise parent respects their right to their own life style. Unfortunately, some parents, especially those who have lost a spouse, try to live for or through their children or grandchildren. This vicarious living causes resentment and guilt feelings.

Most mature children want parents to remain independent. But when necessary, most children will step in to help.

Grandparents can enjoy the little ones. But teens and above, especially boys, aren't interested in grandparents. Grandparents and grandchildren are separated by ideological differences. But if they live together, they're not so prejudiced.

As we age, the sibling role becomes more important. We have memories to share.

Friends

Aerodynamics engineers tell us that as each bird flying

in a V formation flaps its wings, it creates an uplift for the bird behind.

"When a bird falls out of formation he suddenly feels the extra weight of trying to go it alone." Real friends give us a lift like that.[12]

Our early retirement years provide opportunities for us to fellowship with others in our age group. Some of us fortunate golden agers live among those we've known for a long time. Others must move away from familiar surroundings and faces. All of us lose friends through moving or through death. To compensate for this loss, we must make new friends.

We continue to need a sense of individuality and a recognition of our own worth. We need to feel a sense of belonging and being valued by others. Friends provide that.

Widowhood

The specter of widowhood haunts even the most courageous married couple. No matter how hard we try to banish the thought, refusing to think about the possibility will not make it go away. Of course we can never fully prepare for such trauma. Yet we can take certain steps to help us survive.

1. Accept the fact that you really don't know which of you will die first. After his wife died of a heart attack, Henry said, "We always thought I'd go first." Her death caught him completely off guard.

2. Convince yourself ahead of time that you can live without your companion. "I just couldn't live without you" sounds romantic. But "I'd hate to have to live without you" is more practical.

3. Refuse to become dependent on your spouse. After losing her husband, Helen discovered that she had depended on him to drive in heavy traffic and to find their way around in the city. Ruth doesn't drive at all. If her husband dies first, she'll be confined to her home unless she learns to drive.

4. Know your spouse's business. Tom ran his own business for thirty years, owned a number of commercial buildings, and worked for a bank to attract new industry. Despite failing health, he "protected" his wife by taking care of all records and correspondence himself. A few nights before his death, he stayed up late working on his books. Both realized his condition; yet they couldn't discuss financial matters. But after his death, his wife had to cope with all those papers alone. When she needed something, she had to look through a closet full of boxes and files to find it. What had always seemed easy for Tom became a nightmare for her.

The reverse happens if the wife manages the finances and the husband knows nothing about them.

Few couples can discuss business when one is facing death. When Sam realized he had terminal cancer, however, he and Ada talked frankly about her future. With four children under the age of eight, they knew careful planning was vital. They worked together to buy a small farm while he was well. At his suggestion, Ada kept the farm and enough livestock to provide for her and the children. His advice helped her manage alone.

5. Cultivate outside interests. Senior Citizens' centers provide activities to help you keep busy. Volunteering your services to some organization will help pass the time and get you out of the house. A part-time job may help you adjust and give you a feeling of worth.

6. Keep in touch with friends. A few years ago we visited some friends we had known well thirty years ago. But we discovered that, with the exception of a few incidents we all remembered, we had few interests in common. Somehow, when we lose touch with friends, we have less and less to talk about when we do meet.

7. Make up your mind right now that you will, with God's help, find ways to cope with grief when it comes. When Chris lost her husband, she showed little outward emotion. As years passed, she acted as though nothing happened. Yet those of us who knew her and her husband

through thirty years of marriage realize that she misses him very much. Her friends expected her to break under the pressure of suppressed grief. Most people would. But she has held steady. She found a way to cope.

Annette determined that friends wouldn't avoid her because she talked so much about her deceased husband. She controlled her impulse to cry or mention him to her friends.

A year after his wife's death, however, Jim can't mention her name without crying.

Peggy was convinced that God would heal her husband of cancer. When he died, her faith suffered a severe blow. As she wrestled with her problems, her grief persisted. A year dragged by, two years, and more before she could come to terms with her grief.

Somewhere between the extremes of suppressed and overwhelming grief lies the healthy reaction. Some of us need professional help to cope. Not many can handle suppressed grief. For good mental health, a certain amount and period of grieving is important and natural. Yet failure to deal with grief within a reasonable time frame may indicate or cause severe emotional problems. It is vital to get on with our lives.

When a loved one dies, a survivor usually goes through the following stages:

1. *Shock*—This is a frozen or blunted emotional response, and sometimes people think the survivor doesn't care. The mind can't function adequately under emotional stress or during shock and trauma. The mind can handle only a certain amount of information. When a person is in shock, too much confusion will cause the brain to overload and cause one to cry. After losing a spouse or someone else very close, a person should avoid making a life-changing decision for at least a year.

2. *Emotion or tears*—Although family and close friends say, "Don't cry," crying starts the healing process.

3. *Depression and loneliness*—Even though people are around, a person still feels alone and lonely. It is a normal

feeling, but giving in to self-pity can lead to deep depression.

4. *Panic*—A widow may feel panic. To relieve her fears, she needs someone to talk calmly and pray with her.

5. *Guilt*—Every survivor will feel some guilt. Most will feel guilty about someone or something they said.

Twice a widow, my mother must have known about this feeling.

"When I'm gone," she sometimes told me, "don't worry about what you said."

This statement usually came after she and I had a disagreement. She knew that, as a child and young adult, I had a very tender conscience. And she didn't want me to feel bad about what I said, especially to feel guilty after she was gone.

God's forgiveness takes care of real guilt. The false guilt, we must refuse to accept. Most of us do the best we know for those we love. None of us will have perfect performance.

6. *Hostility and resentment*—A widow usually seeks someone to blame. She may blame anyone connected to the situation in which her husband died. She may become bitter toward the physician, God, or even her lost partner. This feeling is normal. But she must deal with it.

On a news broadcast reporting the drowning of his two sons and three grandchildren, a father said, "It was God's doings." As a devoted Christian, he firmly believed and accepted that answer.

For a devout Christian adult who can say that without hostility and resentment, such a philosophy or theology works wonders for the emotions. For an unbeliever or a child, however, that explanation may cause extreme bitterness and rebellion.

No one can really understand or explain all the ramifications of death and certainly God's dealings. Rather than say, "God took my father," it's safer to say, "Cancer or heart attack or accident took my father." Why blame God for things we often bring on ourselves or others bring on us?

We can avoid the hostility by placing the blame where it belongs, then asking God to help us deal with our grief.

7. *Hope*—For the Christian, there is hope in Jesus Christ.

How long will it take to get over the loss? The answer depends on a number of factors: (1) the type of person, the amount of emotion she allows herself or he allows himself to show; the profession she or he follows; (2) the person's relationship with the Lord; (3) family ties; (4) the type of people the person is with. If one is a mature Christian and growing in the Lord, it will take much less time. Helping others will also be a real healing process. Planning something to look forward to also speeds the process.

A widow needs someone with whom to talk about the deceased. Often well-meaning friends and family members try to keep from mentioning the name. Of course, they think failing to talk about the loved one helps the widow to get her mind on other things.

Esther insisted that assumption is false. "Your mind is on your lost loved one all the time anyhow," she said. "Talking with an understanding person who loved him also helps relieve the pressure." After the death of her first husband, that understanding confidante was his mother. Sharing their mutual sorrow brought healing.

As the Bible says, "Bear ye one another's burdens, and so fulfil the law of Christ" (Gal. 6:2).

Dating

After a period of grieving, a surviving spouse often starts looking for someone to date. The waiting period varies according to how long friends think is long enough, how long the survivor has known the one he or she plans to date, and whether the survivor is a man or a woman.

Many couples date for companionship only. They may enjoy each other's company. They go out to eat. They may go on cruises or tours with others their age. But they may prefer to remain "faithful" to a deceased companion. Some of these couples date for years with no thought of marriage.

Other couples date with marriage in mind. They may agree to wait for a period of time for "getting over" a lost mate. But they plan to marry eventually.

Unfortunately, for widows who want to date, the few eligible men pass them by like a hummingbird passes an onion patch. For reasons of their own, men often prefer younger women. This preference, coupled with the oversupply of widows and social disapproval of assertive women, discourages older ladies from entering the competition.

"I'd rather smell perfume than liniment any time," explained one widower when asked why he married a woman half his age.

In a letter to "Dear Abby," a lady in her 60's complained that eligible men are too busy "fishing, hunting, and playing the field" until their health is threatened. Then they start looking in earnest for a woman to take care of them. Some, she claimed, had even asked her how high her blood pressure was.

When a man suddenly becomes interested in her as soon as he gets an unfavorable diagnosis, she suggests that he look for a retirement home like she plans to do when she needs care.

"Dear Abby" was speechless. I wonder why.

Evidently that lady is like another widow who told potential suitors: "I'll do well to take care of myself from here on."

For whatever reasons, of the 6 million widows in this country, only 1 out of 7 will remarry.

Relieved to find a listener, a friend brought up the subject of his deceased wife and of his dating.

"She's a nice woman," he said of his lady friend. "I enjoy her company. But I don't have any real feeling for her."

He certainly didn't owe me an explanation. But he needed a sounding board so he could examine his own feelings and ideas. Aware that I knew his first wife, he talked about her, reminiscing about their courtship and marriage.

"Gradually," he said, "Jewel is beginning to fade just a little each day."

Before ending the conversation, however, he said, "I fell in love with her the day I met her. And I'm still in love with her."

When I mentioned this statement to a friend who has remarried, tears came to her eyes. I think she knows the feeling.

As long as one wrestles with such feelings, it's hardly fair to a new spouse for him or her to remarry.

The late Dorothy Dix wrote that no woman is good enough to compete with one who has been dead long enough to become perfect. That goes for a man, too.

Remarriage

A retired couple were discussing some friends who had just remarried.

"If I should die," the husband began, "I suppose you'd get married again."

"Yes," his wife agreed. "I probably would."

"And this guy would eat at my place at the table?"

"Yes."

"He'd sleep in my bed?"

"Yes."

"He'd sit in my recliner?"

"Yes."

"And he'd play golf with my clubs?"

"Oh, no!" she said.

"Why not?"

"Oh, he's left-handed," she explained.

Even if the proposed next spouse hasn't been chosen, the subject remains practically out of bounds for any couple.

Unfortunately, some husbands or wives insist that their spouse promise not to remarry. Some break such a promise and suffer guilt feelings as a result.

Surely all any wife or husband can reasonably demand is that a spouse live up to the marriage vows, give the deceased a respectable period of grief, and not make a fool of himself or herself.

Remarriage includes certain basic problems. A couple needs common interests, a good sense of humor, ability to get along with others, communication skills, reasonable health, financial resources, and a willingness to adapt. Love differs somewhat in an older marriage or remarriage. Yet it still plays a vital role.

When one or both partners have children, a remarriage can cause a tremendous strain on relationships. If money is involved or if children want certain possessions that belonged to a deceased parent, they may cause trouble.

Before remarriage, a couple should discuss all possible problem situations and agree on solutions.

June and Fred have what looks like an ideal remarriage. His children and hers condoned the marriage. Everyone is happy for them. But Fred brought more money into the marriage than did June. Now he insists that his money should go to his children.

Jim and Marie married after several years of courtship. He set aside a specified amount of money for his children. They live on the rest of his income. Living in her home bought with money from her first husband's estate, they enjoy the benefits of both incomes and yet provide for their children.

Grace married a man twenty years her senior. He spent his last two years bedfast at home and in a nursing home. Grace cared for him at home. For a year, she went every day to feed him and take care of his personal needs in the nursing home. When he died, his children complained about the amount of money she got from his will.

In addition to money, children often cause trouble because of jealousy or mere preconceived notions of what is best for their parent. Preparing ahead of time can avoid most such confrontations.

Despite the problems, remarriage with the right person

makes life much more rewarding at any age, even in later years. The right person will likely be a well-adjusted and financially independent individual, someone you've known a long time, one whom your children approve.

Chapter 6
Church Avenue: Spiritual Development

Leaving the college, we turn onto Church Avenue. You will notice that Golden Acres Cathedral dominates this lovely area. In addition to providing for the spiritual development of the community, the church offers opportunities for social enrichment as well.

If we hurry, we should find a seat in time for the worship service.

Message of Hope

Good. We made it in time for the music. Let's sit near the entrance.

The white-haired gentleman leading the congregational singing is Bryan. His enthusiasm for old hymns and gospel songs is contagious.

Coming to the platform now are Dr. and Mrs. Howard Walker. Before retirement, they taught in college. He sings solos and she accompanies him at the piano. They use their talents in the local church and in revivals across the country.

Our organist, Beth, is a retired college professor. Recently remarried, she and her husband have just come home from an overseas teaching assignment.

Our guest minister today is Dr. Victor Wheeler, a former seminary professor. Besides teaching a course at the college, he preaches in revivals and special services.

I'll keep quiet now. You won't want to miss a word of his message.

Faith That Removes Mountains

"No doubt King Jehoshaphat of Judah remembered

such examples as Caleb when a multitude of Ammonites came against God's people. In Second Chronicles, chapter 20, we read this story:

"'And Jehoshaphat feared, and set himself to seek the LORD' (v. 3).

"Gathering his people into God's house, he prayed:

'... O LORD God of our fathers, *art* not thou God... and rulest *not* thou over all the kingdoms of the heathen? and in thine hand *is there not* power and might, so that none is able to withstand thee? *Art* not thou our God, *who* didst drive out the inhabitants of this land before thy people Israel, and gavest it to the seed of Abraham thy friend for ever?' (vs. 6, 7).

"Jehoshaphat reminds God of His faithfulness to answer when His people cry unto Him. Most prayers are self-centered, but not this one. The king's prayer (vs. 6-12) is God-centered, not problem-centered.

"He continues, '... We have no might against this great company that cometh against us; neither know we what to do: but our eyes *are* upon thee' (v. 12).

"God's answer: 'Be not afraid nor dismayed by reason of this great multitude; for the battle *is* not yours but God's' (v. 15).

"'Ye shall not *need* to fight in this *battle*,' God adds. 'Set yourselves, stand ye *still*, and see the salvation of the LORD with you, O Judah and Jerusalem: fear not, nor be dismayed; tomorrow go out against them: for the LORD *will* be with you' (v. 17).

"The problem is not yours, but God's. Oh, that we could get that through our heads! We waste so much time and energy behaving as though it's our problem.

"In the old favorite song 'What a Friend,' the poet reminds us of the peace we forfeit and the pain we bear when we fail to turn to God for solutions to problems.

"Following the example of his predecessors, however, King Jehoshaphat knew how to cope. After praying and reminding God that this was His problem, the king trusted God's reply.

"With hordes of enemy troups advancing toward the little swarm of 'grasshoppers,' Jehoshaphat called his people to worship. He asked the choir to sing. Standing in front of those terrified soldiers, the choir sang the king's request: 'Praise the LORD; for his mercy *endureth* for ever' (v. 21).

"While His people worshiped, the Lord 'set ambushments against the children of Ammon, Moab, and Mount Seir, which were come against Judah; and they were smitten' (v. 22). In fact, they turned on each other.

"The historical books of the Old Testament report many such events. God delivered His people when they turned to Him for help.

"The New Testament emphasizes God's love and care for the individual. It reveals a loving Father, willing to forgive and to provide for every need. He's the Christian's burden-bearer and strong defense."

Fellowship

If we can make our way through the aisles, with all these people congregating to visit, we'll look in on several Sunday School classes. In these close-knit groups, members share everything from news of the birth of a great-grandchild to prayer requests for family and friends. The class has common concerns and interests. This is truly a fellowship of the saints.

Service

As we walk through the halls, you'll see what makes this church tick—the volunteers.

From ushers Norman and Fred in the auditorium to eighty-three-year old Sarah who works in her Sunday School class—scores of volunteers make up the team.

Sunday School teachers include: Rev. L. E. Thomas, Professor Grace Hankins, Missionary Opal Stiverson, Administrator Charles Coppock, Businessmen Herman

Thompkins and G. W. Price.
Visitors in hospitals and nursing homes include: Rev. D. S. Moore, George Franklin, and James Hensley.

The business of the church requires another crew to serve on boards and committees. Many of our retirees devote a considerable amount of time and energy to church business.

Other volunteers serve behind the scenes with little public recognition.

One whose work is highly visible is Brother Short. A former postal employee, now nearing eighty-six, he works several days each week beautifying the church lawn.

Once he resigned, but as soon as he could tactfully do so, he resumed the job. One glance at the lush, immaculate lawn answers the question "Why?" He's using his special gift and expertise in horticulture to the glory of God.

Whether it's Brother Short pruning a shrub, Ruth Jones serving a dinner, or Jane Brannon making coffee for the choir—service is the key to church growth.

God enables these Christians and many others to continue serving Him with their gifts long after their retirement.

Without the help of volunteers, the church could not function. But with everyone giving time, energy, and expertise for its advancement, the church serves the spiritual needs of its community.

Activity

Speaking of social activities earlier, I mentioned that our church sponsors a dinner each month, Sunday School class parties, and small-group get-togethers.

We'll move on to our recreation center, where many of these activities take place. You'll notice, we have kitchen facilities, with a stove, sink, and refrigerator. We have adequate space, tables and chairs, a piano, and a fireplace.

Most of our dinners are potluck. A few are catered. Ladies with a flair for decorating bring centerpieces for tables. Others help with serving and cleaning up.

For small groups, we have a number of good eating places within easy driving distance of the church. Our people enjoy eating out with friends. A few invite friends home for dinner or refreshments.

Providing wholesome activity for its members plays a vital role in our Golden Acres church program.

And, lest you think all we do is eat, let me tell you about our travels.

Travel

If we come by here about seven o'clock tomorrow morning, we'll see chartered buses parked in front of this building. Senior adults from the church will be loading suitcases and boarding buses.

The SAMS (Senior Adult Ministeries) trips have taken this group east, west, north, and south. They have covered most of the United States and some other places.

Tomorrow the group is headed for the annual Golden Agers retreat. Everyone looks forward to this week of recreation, social fellowship, and spiritual enrichment.

A smaller group has just returned from a church-sponsored cruise outside our country.

For international church assemblies, our local church reserves a block of rooms and airline seats for its senior adults.

A few retirees have participated in Work and Witness teams, donating their time and energy to helping build a church on a mission field.

All these church-sponsored travel opportunities keep us on the go as much as we want to be gone.

Family Relationship

Our pastor often refers to the congregation as a part of the great family of God. In our fellowship, we feel a spirit of kinship in a very special way. We have probably lost parents, brothers, and sisters. To experience family ties, we senior adults must "adopt" parents and siblings from the congregation. With them we share as we used to share with our own family.

Even when relatives are still living, our values and life styles often differ. Non-Christians don't have the same interests as Christians have. It's only natural that a fellow Christian often seems closer than members of your own family.

From its earliest days, the Christian church enjoyed a family relationship. Words spoken of the early church, "Behold how they love one another," still characterize genuine believers. "Let brotherly love continue" (Heb. 13:1) makes a good motto for all Christians.

Although most of us no longer call church friends "Brother" or "Sister," we still sense the family relationship within the church.

Learning Opportunities

The Apostle Paul wrote: "Study to shew thyself approved unto God, a workman that needeth not to be ashamed, rightly dividing the word of truth" (2 Tim. 2:15).

To encourage spiritual growth and intellectual understanding, our church makes available to its members a number of learning opportunities.

Periodic prayer seminars teach us how to pray more effectively.

Most members attend Sunday School classes on Sunday. There they concentrate on a portion of Scripture. Sometimes they discuss the lesson. More often they listen to a lecture by a qualified teacher. They usually get a "takeaway" truth to apply to daily living.

For those interested in in-depth study of the Bible, the church trains teachers and schedules classes. These meet one night each week for seven-week periods. They cover both the Old and New Testaments.

Small groups of ladies meet one day each week for Bible

study. They concentrate on a book or a theme from Scripture.

Self-Fulfillment

Under the auspices of the church, everyone is encouraged to strive for self-fulfillment.

Through a message of hope, we learn that God has a plan for our lives.

In fellowship with other Christians, we sense that we are not alone.

In service, we can use our God-given talents for their intended purpose.

Through our activities and travels, we share our joys and excitement.

Within the church family, we find a kinship to enrich our lives.

By our learning opportunities, we better prepare ourselves for realizing our spiritual potential.

All of these benefits provide the soil for personal growth and self-fulfillment.

Thank God for the church.

Chapter 7
Commerce Drive: Money Management Resources

Now that we've visited the church and its senior adult facilities, it's time to board the bus again and head for Commerce Drive.

Whatever our financial situation, we're all interested in managing money efficiently. "Will my money last as long as I do?" is a question of concern to most of us. Before we join the throng in search of advice at the bank, the attorney's office, and the automobile agency, let's stop and consider God's financial principles.

As our loving Heavenly Father, God never intended us to suffer the humiliation, guilt, and remorse inherent in financial disaster. By practicing His principles, we can avoid most economic woes.

I. We will tithe on a regular basis: Through His prophet, God commands: "Bring ye all the tithes into the storehouse, that there may be meat in mine house, and prove me now herewith, saith the LORD of hosts, if I will not open you the windows of heaven, and pour you out a blessing, that *there shall* not *be room* enough *to receive it"* (Mal. 3:10).

Before she ever heard a sermon on tithing, Esther read Malachi and an article on the subject. A widow with four small children, she began practicing and talking about tithing.

"You can't outgive God," she often said.

A few weeks before her death, she took a tour of her new church in a wheel chair. Looking at all the splendor around her, she said, "You know, I helped build this church with my tithe."

"You surely did," I assured her.

Little as it was, her tithe belonged to God and Esther

enjoyed paying it.

Jesus had more to say about man and his relationship to money than about any other moral question. In fact, two-thirds of his parables deal with money. He warns: "You cannot serve two masters; God and money. For you will hate one and love the other, or else the other way around" (Matt. 6:24 TLB).

II. We will save a part of all we earn. King Solomon tells us to consider the ant and save. He adds: "The wise man saves for the future, but the foolish man spends whatever he gets" (Prov. 21:20 TLB).*

One pastor's advice: "Pay God ten percent, save ten percent, and live on the rest."

III. We will anticipate needs and plan ahead to meet them. "Any enterprise," observes King Solomon, "is built by wise planning, becomes strong through common sense, and profits wonderfully by keeping abreast of the facts" (Prov. 24:3,4 TLB).

We tend to reason that "barring unforeseen circumstances" we can make it. But no way can we "bar unforeseen circumstances." "How do you know what's going to happen tomorrow?" James asks (James 4:14 TLB).

IV. We will provide for a minimum amount of insurance coverage. According to King Solomon: "A prudent man foresees difficulties ahead and prepares for them; the simpleton goes blindly on and suffers the consequences" (Prov. 22:3 TLB).

Since no one knows exactly how much coverage he needs, each must decide how much or how little is the minimum.

V. We will not countersign for another person's loan unless necessary to meet a need in our immediate family. "Unless you have the extra cash on hand," warns Solomon, "don't countersign a note. Why risk everything you own? They'll even take your bed!" (Prov. 22:26, 27 TLB). He adds: "He who gives surety for a stranger will smart

---

*Verses marked TLB are taken from *The Living Bible*, copyright 1971 by Tyndale House Publishers, Wheaton, IL. Used by permission.

for it, but he who hates suretyship is secure" (Prov. 11:15). He calls it "poor judgment" (Prov. 17:18 TLB). Enough said.

VI. We will not purchase on a time payment plan any of the following: food, clothing, gasoline, vacation, any item of luxury, any item for pleasure or recreation. The Apostle John declares: "... The ambition to buy everything that appeals to you, and the pride that comes from wealth and importance—these are not from God" (1 John 2:16b TLB). "Just as the rich rule the poor," Solomon notes, "so the borrower is servant to the lender" (Prov. 22:7 TLB).

VII. We will pay all financial obligations on or before the date due. "Don't withhold payment of your debts," Solomon says. "Don't say, 'some other time,' if you can pay now" (Prov. 3:27 TLB).

When Frank bought his new car last year, he called Mr. Walker, president of his bank, and said, "I've found a new car I want to buy. I'll need a loan for $4,000."

"Go ahead and write the check," Mr. Walker said. "Then come in and sign the papers. Your wife can sign next time she comes in."

Does Mr. Walker automatically say that to anyone who wants a loan? Hardly. If he were that careless, his bank would fail like many others.

But Frank and his wife have established a good track record. They once owed that bank over $20,000 on a small business. When the business failed to prosper, they could have filed for bankruptcy. Instead, they sold the business, got a job, and repaid the loan ahead of time. Now they can face Mr. Walker and talk as an equal. If they need a loan or financial advice, they can get it from him.

VIII. We will not participate in any get-rich-quick schemes, such as pyramid plans, chain letters, small, closely held corporations whose management has no history of sound, productive results. Again, the wise man says: "Steady plodding brings prosperity, hasty speculation brings poverty" (Prov. 21:5 TLB). "Trying to get rich quick is evil and leads to poverty" (Prov. 28:22 TLB). "The naive believe everything, but the prudent man considers his steps" (Prov. 14:15 TLB). "What a shame—yes, how stupid!—to decide before knowing all the facts" (Prov. 18:13 TLB).

IX. As God provides, we will set aside a portion of our earnings to enable us to minister to the needs about us as God reveals them, giving cash only on condition that the recipient receive counsel.

The Apostle Paul says: "They (who have of this world's goods) are to do good, to be rich in good deeds; liberal and generous, thus laying up for themselves a good foundation for the future, so that they may take hold of the life that is indeed" (1 Tim. 6:18,19 TLB). "When you help the poor," Solomon says, "you are lending to the Lord—and He pays wonderful interest on your loan" (Prov. 19:17 TLB).

"Before I give money to a stranger," the late Dr. E. S. Phillips used to say, "I insist on praying with that person."

By giving to reputable organizations only, we can rest assured of accountability.

Paul Harvey warned us as early as December 22, 1984, that our aid to Ethiopia was "being diverted by the Marxist government for political purposes." He said that, "blinded by tears, American churchmen were overrunning their headlights." Money sent to relieve hunger has been used for "relocation" of Ethiopian farmers in a program "closely akin to roundups of Jews in Nazi Germany." Such "'relocation' has claimed 100,000 lives." Existing in unbelievably inhumane conditions, political enemies of the Marxist regime suffer agony because our money rewarded the government.

"*The Wall Street Journal,*" says Harvey, "which has tried for most of a year to ventilate this stench, reports the added horror that 'it would not be possible except for the aid and silence of western relief officials.'" "The resettlement camps of Ethiopia are Buchenwald in everything but the ovens," he adds.[1]

No doubt those who solicited and those who contributed firmly believed the money would go to feed the hungry.

Evidently only that actually distributed personally by missionaries and native Christian workers reached the starving. The rest only increased their suffering. We can trust our local and general church to use our offerings for their intended purpose.

X. Our goal will be contentment with what God has given us. Discontentment results in covetousness and greed. The writer to the Hebrews admonishes us: "Keep your life free from the love of money and be content with what you have; for he has said, 'I will never fail you nor forsake you'" (Heb. 13:5 TLB). Paul wrote to the Philippian church: "For I have learned in whatever state I am, to be content" (Phil. 4:11b TLB).

Though contrary to the spirit of our age, God's financial principles are valid today. By following His guidelines, we can live more solvent, serene, and satisfied lives. Without the harassment of creditors, the anxiety of unwise investments, and the pangs of a guilty conscience, we can exert a greater influence for God. We can rest assured of His continued presence and provision.

With God's counsel fresh in our minds, let's learn what we can from other sources.

First Citizens Bank of Golden Acres

Except for the age of its customers, this bank is like any other one. Since it caters to senior adults, we can learn a lot here.

First, we need to fill out a questionnaire.

QUESTIONNAIRE

MONTHLY INCOME

Social Security	_____
Pension	_____
Annuity	_____
Stock Dividends	_____
Interest	_____
Rent	_____
Salary	_____
Other	_____
Total	_____

MONTHLY PAYMENTS

Home Mortgage	_____
Automobile	_____
Bank Loan	_____
Credit Card	_____
Other	_____
Total	_____

MONTHLY LIVING EXPENSES

Food	_____	Medical	_____
Rent	_____	Books, etc.	_____
Utilities	_____	Travel	_____
Clothing	_____	Entertainment	_____
Insurance	_____	Church	_____
Taxes	_____	Personal items	_____
Other	_____	Other	_____
		Total	_____

Your financial profile gives you an idea of where you stand. If your income exceeds your expenditures, you can relax and maybe carry over part of the excess. If the two columns are about the same, you have cause for concern. And, obviously, if your expenses exceed your income, you're already in trouble. It's time to take a serious look at possible alternatives. But let's hope you're in the first category.

Suppose your monthly income exceeds your expenses by $500. You'd like to invest that money. Through TV and newspaper advertising and through your junk mail, you're aware of investment options. You'd like to know which is best for you.

Unfortunately, in a dog-eat-dog economic society, it's virtually impossible to find an unbiased opinion. And the complexity of finance sometimes requires professional counseling to determine what is best for an individual investor. A consultant may be well worth his or her fee.

But, to keep it simple, let's look at a few basics.

Real Estate

You're watching TV. A commercial comes on. A millionaire will conduct a seminar in your city and tell you how to make a fortune buying real estate with little or no equity.

Maybe you invest in a book on how to make a million dollars in real estate.

The theory implies that once you get started, you can use one piece of property as collateral for money borrowed to buy the next. Thus, you can keep increasing your holdings indefinitely. In record time, you can be a millionaire—on paper, at least.

I know a lady who paid the tuition and attended a seminar advertised on TV. She swallowed the theory hook, line, and sinker. She and her husband bought an old house to remodel. They moved from their lovely show place to the ancient two-story in a run-down neighborhood.

As they remodeled, they collected rent from their former home. While they fixed up an old house, someone else enjoyed their nice one.

But they kept buying junky houses and renting them to junky tenants. Collecting rent caused major problems.

Despite the headaches—including costly court battles—rental property can be an excellent investment for one who doesn't get carried away.

With its depreciation, expense, and interest deduction, rental property makes a good tax shelter. And, with the right tenants, it's a good source of income. Most important, it usually appreciates in value. For example, a house that sold for $30,000 ten years ago may sell for $90,000 or more today, depending on its location and condition, and, of course, the market.

Investment in real estate may be limited to property with capital gains potential. If conditions are right and if you can afford to wait while the value of the property escalates, you may reap substantial dividends.

While real estate has its risks, it has its rewards as well.

Bank Securities

Certificates of Deposit, Money Market Funds, Individual Retirement Accounts, and Treasury Bills experienced a hey-day while interest rates remained above 10%. Even with lower interest rates and less-attractive tax incentives, IRA's continue to lure investors. And at 5 to 6 percent, other securities maintain their popularity among investors demanding government secured investments.

If you're tempted to invest with a financial institution advertising interest or dividend rates considerably higher than the average, investigate. In general, the higher the rate, the more risky the venture. Read the fine print. Usually you'll notice "not guaranteed by any government agency" or a similar statement at the end of an advertisement of high rates. Beware!

For its members, the American Association of Retired Persons provides a number of investment opportunities at higher-than-average earnings potential. Their Liberty Account Funds and their Scudder Funds offer a variety of options.

Stocks and Bonds

A number of the AARP investment funds involve stocks and bonds. The American Leaders Fund, Inc., for example, invests in U.S. Government bonds and Corporate bonds and more than thirty stocks. Their rate of earnings led me to transfer money from one account into that one. Incidentally, you can make arrangements to transfer money via telephone from one fund to another within a group of funds.

Of course you have various options available in the stocks and bonds market. Scores of brokers advertise their readiness to help you make decisions. The problem is finding one you feel like trusting with your money.

Annuities

If you start in time and don't mind losing control over your assets, annuities may be for you. You have a number of options. You can pay into the annuity over a period of years, with the assurance that you and perhaps your spouse will receive a specified amount each month after retirement. In some cases, the company gets to keep what is left in case you and your spouse die before the money is used up.

Some retirees invest in annuities to be sure of a steady monthly income in their last years.

If you want to keep control of your money, however, you might prefer other investments.

Other

The list of opportunities is endless: Gold, Art, Jewelry, Part-time business, Money lending—almost anything, in fact, has money-making potential.

Even $500 per month, if invested regularly and wisely, will increase substantially within a few years.

If your financial profile shows that your income and expenditures are about the same, you need to consider ways to improve your standing.

And if your expenditures exceed your income, you're in trouble. It's time to take a serious look at possible solutions.

1. You can increase your income. If you have good health, job skills, and experience, you should have no trouble finding work. Many retirees do. You might be happier working in a different kind of job, especially if you retired because of burnout or stress. A hobby could provide a source of income.

If you're a retired teacher, you have a number of options. You can advertise for students to tutor. You can sign up for substitute teaching. It's a rough life, but it pays well. You might apply to teach night classes at a nearby college. If you're an elementary teacher, Day-Care Centers desperately need your expertise.

Secretarial, sales, and domestic jobs provide part-time opportunities. Carpenters and mechanics can work for others or for themselves. One electrician says he keeps busier than ever since he retired. No doubt many others share that experience.

A dozen or so men from here like to drive. They make themselves available to local automobile dealers. If one doesn't have the car his customer wants, he can use his computer to locate it. Once he finds it, he can either arrange a dealer trade or buy it. He calls a man from his list of drivers to go after it. If he needs several drivers, he may send them in a van to drive the cars back. Every town has car dealers. But if you really need money, this job isn't for you. It's entirely too spasmodic.

The list of part-time jobs is endless. The Classified Ad section of a typical metropolitan newspaper suggests scores of possibilities. You should be able to find one that provides extra income without lowering your dignity.

2. *You can dip into your savings*—if you have any. Those of us who lived through the Great Depression—and what retiree didn't—tend to consider savings as sacred. What we have managed to accummulate across the years must remain untouched, even if it's buried in the back yard. It is there to be used only in case of extreme emergency.

Of course it's always wise to have some savings for a rainy day. But, considering the effect of inflation on the value of our savings, unless they're invested where they'll earn a substantial dividend, maybe it isn't such a bad idea to dip into them.

Suppose, for example, you've managed to save $25,000. You've invested $15,000 in IRA's, $5,000 in Money Market

Certificates, and $5,000 in stocks. If you're in a high tax bracket, possibly your IRA's will continue to pay off. At a mere 5 or 5.5%, however, your Money Market Certificates are barely keeping ahead of inflation. Your stocks? Well it all depends.

You might find a better use for some of your money.

3. You can reduce your expenditures. After you retire, you will notice some expenses automatically decrease.

You probably won't need so many clothes. Those you have will last longer. And you won't need to have them cleaned so often.

Your car expenses will likely decrease. That is, unless you travel more.

If you prepare more meals at home, your food costs will diminish. Many retirees, however, prefer to eat out and pay the extra. If you live near a fast food place, you can compromise by bringing part of the meal home and supplementing with a drink and dessert.

Spending more time in bed should decrease your fuel bills. Since most people need more heat and less air conditioning as they get older, utility costs will vary. Closing unused rooms and closets helps cut the cost of heating and cooling.

Other expenses may increase. When you retired, you probably lost your group hospital or health insurance coverage. If you're not old enough for Medicare, your health insurance will take a huge bite out of your monthly budget. Even with Medicare, most of us need a supplemental health policy.

A friend who visited me in the hospital after my cancer surgery called a few days later to discuss my symptoms and compare them with hers. She had some of the same problems. I urged her to see her doctor.

"Oh, I couldn't have an operation," she said. "I don't have any insurance except Medicare."

She didn't have the surgery. Maybe she didn't need it. She's still alive after five years.

But it's sad to need medical treatment and not be able to

afford it. And we need more care as we age.

Before entering the hospital, I asked a friend—a vice-president of a large insurance company—to examine my policies. He assured me that all I had to worry about was getting well. I'm convinced that made a difference in my amazing progress.

Many major insurance companies offer Medicare supplemental health insurance. By comparing costs and provisions, you can find a policy that fits your needs. When you find such a plan, you may want to cancel some present policies to avoid duplicate coverage.

Some HMO (Health Maintenance Organization) plans cover almost everything, even most of the cost for prescription drugs. My husband and I tried an HMO plan for a year. We enjoyed walking out of a doctor's office with no bill. But when my ophthalmologist refused to accept assignment, my doctor withdrew from the plan, and a supplier reported difficulty in collecting for medical supplies, we cancelled. There are, however, reputable HMO's.

Anything you can do to reduce costs and maintain peace of mind is certainly worth the effort.

Expenses for social activities, entertainment, leisure, and recreation may increase after retirement. You may enjoy inviting friends over for dinner or a snack. You may attend more cultural events. You'll probably spend more on reading material. You may buy recreational equipment and spend more on travel. Now that you have time for such luxuries, you feel entitled to them. After all, you've worked hard. You deserve a break.

Live it up! Why not? It's yours to decide.

Having just mailed a check for automobile insurance, I'm reminded of another big chunk of the monthly budget. Paying home insurance hurts less because it's part of our house payment. Life insurance premiums took their toll on the budget until we arranged for paid-up insurance.

Shopping for home and automobile insurance this year saved money for us. Careful evaluation of our life insurance policies in the light of our present needs led us to make changes. We had already taken a loan at 5% interest several years earlier. When Money Market certificates were bringing in 14% interest, we considered borrowing on our life insurance policies to invest. We withdrew our request upon learning that we'd be required to surrender our policies to get all the loan value. Finally we took paid-up insurance.

Contributions to charitable organizations, gifts for showers and other occasions, personal items—all add up, often throwing the budget off balance.

"Youth," someone has said, "is concerned with sex; middle age, with ambition; old age, with money."

Most of us are primarily concerned with making our money last as long as we do.

If you can't or don't want to increase your income or reduce your expenditures, you may have a desirable option.

4. You may invade your capital assets.

Even if you have no money in savings, you probably have considerable equity in your home. Aside from a loved one or health, the last thing you want to lose is your home. You don't want to think of losing it. But read on. You may be able to "have your cake and eat it too." A variety of home equity conversion plans can enable you to live in your home while using your equity.

a. Reverse mortgage

Some companies will loan you up to 80%—some even more—of your home's appraised value. They can arrange to pay you the loan in monthly installments over a specified period—maybe eight to ten years. The company may pay the taxes and insurance, or you may pay them.

At the end of the time period, the principle and interest must be repaid. By that time, however, the home will likely be worth more—maybe enough to renegotiate a loan.

If you can't repay the loan on the date specified, you must sell the home to pay the debt. Should you die before that date, the house will be sold to repay the debt. Your estate, however, gets the remaining profits, if any.

Variations of this basic arrangement include one providing for you to remain in your home and receive monthly payments as long as you live in the house.

b. Shared appreciation reverse mortgage

In this arrangement, the lender shares in the increased value of the home. The open-ended loan is not repaid until the house sells. This plan is a gamble on long life.

c. Sale-leaseback contract

This arrangement provides for a buyer to pay 70 to 85% of the appraised value with a guarantee that you can live in the house as long as you want to. The buyer pays 10% down and the rest in installments over a period of years based on the seller's life expectancy.

A lease agreeement is drawn up in which you become a renter. If you move, you will continue to receive your payments. If you die, your estate will get the payments.

The main problem is that you may outlive the period specified. To alleviate this problem, you could arrange for an annuity so the payments would go on until your death.[2]

Before signing a contract, consult your attorney.

Attorney's Office

One of the most important counselors on our money management team is our attorney. We'll stop by his office for suggestions for planning the future, taking advantage of tax breaks, and avoiding financial tangles.

Will and Estate Planning

It may surprise you to learn that hundreds of people who wouldn't think of going without medical, auto, and life insurance have not made a will. They're not taking advantage of the cheapest kind of insurance—a valid will. If they've even thought about one, maybe they've written a few items and names on a piece of notebook paper and called it a will.

I heard about a man who had been bitten by a dog. The

dog was killed and its head sent to the lab. A few days later, friends gathered to break the sad news: The dog was mad.

The threatened man jumped up and ran to his desk. He grabbed a sheet of paper and a pencil and started writing furiously.

"Just a minute," a friend said. "We're going to do everything possible to save your life. Don't start now to make your will."

"Will nothing," the man snapped. "I'm making a list of the people I want to bite!"

It's all right to use an envelope to write a list of those you want to attack. But the homemade will may not be worth the paper you wrote it on to protect the interests of those you love.

Whether you neglect drawing up a will because you don't have very much, you don't care who gets what, or you don't want to think about death, your failure to provide for the distribution of your assets causes unnecessary hardship for survivors.

A highly successful man, an educated man, and a devoted husband and father neglected to make a will. One night he was killed instantly in a car accident. His estate was administered by the courts. According to the state law, his wife was required to report to the court on how she spent every dime of their children's part of the estate. Even so, that family was fortunate in that they received the money—except for exorbitant legal costs.

Others haven't been so lucky.

Drawing up a will is an essential part of family estate planning. Your lawyer plays an important role in each planning procedure. The purpose, of course, is to organize your financial and property matters for your security now and for the security of your family after your death.

To preserve as much of your assets as possible for your survivors, your attorney will discuss estate and gift taxes with you. He may recommend that you set up a trust fund for your spouse and possibly for others such as children or grandchildren. A trust fund for your spouse, for example, may eliminate the risk of excessive taxation as the property passes to children and grandchildren. Such trusts are often used as tax-saving devices.

Trust funds can be used for other purposes as well. A grandmother, for example, wants to set up a trust for her grandchild's college education. A mother doesn't approve of her daughter's spendthrift attitude but wants to be sure that daughter has something to live on in later years. A trust can provide for that need. Your lawyer can give you advice for your particular situation.

Personal Documents

Until a few weeks ago I considered myself well organized. But after reading an article and answering several questions, I wasn't so sure. According to the test results, I'm a borderline case.

Before you criticize me, let me ask you a few questions. Do you ever have to search for an important document? How long would it take for you to lay hands on your last income tax return? Your birth certificate? Your car title? Your home insurance policy?

Maybe you know where to find these papers, but does your spouse?

Obviously both of you should know where to find them and other documents. Someone else should know as well.

Your attorney files a copy of your will and other legal papers he draws up for you. If you don't have a safety deposit box at your bank, your home insurance agent should keep a copy of itemized possessions you keep in the home and pictures taken in each room of your house. In case of fire, someone somewhere outside the home should have access to important documents.

Property Ownership

Joint ownership of your home, car, bank account(s), and securities doesn't mean you don't need a will. It doesn't take care of such matters as final expenses, taxes, and administration of your estate. It demands that your surviving joint tenant deal with business at a traumatic time. It doesn't provide for the possibility that you and the co-owner could be killed in the same accident. In that case, your property might go to the last person you'd want to get it.

On the other hand, joint ownership has its advantages. With a will to supersede it, of course. At your death, the property automatically goes to the surviving co-owner. This transfer requires no taxes and no probate. It may well be the best arrangement. Your lawyer can tell you whether it's best for your individual situation.

If you're considering remarriage, your attorney can draw up an agreement for the distribution of assets among survivors according to the wishes of you and your spouse-to-be. Such a contract, however, does not supersede a will.

Following the advice of a good lawyer can save you anxiety as well as money. Whether your estate be large or small, he can help you preserve it for those you select.

Golden Acres Automobile Agency

America's romance with the automobile by no means ends at 55. Many people buy a "retirement" car. Often it's a luxury model they've never been able to afford. "This one should last us the rest of our lives," they rationalize.

It may last as long as they "need" a car, but those of us who get car fever periodically like a change.

Mr. and Mrs. Jed Johnson rode around town in their late-model panel truck until they were past ninety. Of course, he got a few tickets for minor traffic violations—but who doesn't?

When the new cars came out one fall, Jed got car fever. At a local dealership, he selected a very expensive model and wrote a check for it. The salesman promised delivery that evening.

When Fred heard about the deal, he went straight to the

dealer. Explaining that his 91-year-old father had no business buying a new car, Fred insisted that the deal be cancelled.

Lest the dealer fail to comply, Fred went to his parents' home. Nobody mentioned the car. But as they talked, the old gentleman fidgeted. Finally he suggested that it was time for Fred to leave for prayer meeting.

Fred contrived an excuse and stayed until he was convinced the car wouldn't be delivered.

If you're in the market for a car or you'd like to know more about taking care of the one you have, you should find the following tips helpful.

Buying a Car

1. Be honest with the salesman.
2. Tell him exactly what you want.
3. Tell him what you can afford.
4. Buy from a local dealer.
5. Don't always look for the cheapest price tag.
6. Put your trade-in in the best possible condition.

Keeping Your Car in Top Condition

1. Remove grime regularly.
2. Have your car washed and polished to guard against corrosion.
3. Prevent premature engine and chassis wear by following your Owner's Manual's recommendations for oil filter change and chassis lubrication.
4. Follow suggestions in your Owner's Manual concerning wheel alignment and balancing and rotating tires.
5. Check brakes carefully every 10,000 miles—more often if your driving requires frequent braking or fast stops. Have a brake repair specialist perform this check.
6. Keep lights and windshield wipers in good working order.
7. Visit a radiator repair shop regularly for a check of the cooling system—hose connections, water pump,

gaskets, and all belts.

8. Have your transmission checked periodically. Your local transmission specialist's services include adjustment of bands, change of transmission oil, clean screen, installation of new pan gasket, set transmission linkage, and road test.

9. Keep your car free from rust spots and dents. This service can add years to the life of your car. It's a good idea to buy paint to match your new car; then you can touch up those dents to keep your car looking new and rust free.

10. Have an auto air conditioning specialist check your air conditioning at least once a year.

11. Follow recommendations in your Owner's Manual for engine tune-ups.

Handling Emergencies

1. Starting problems

a. If the battery still has power, press the gas pedal to the floor and then release it. Then turn on the ignition. If it still won't start, pump the gas pedal several times and then try. If there's an odor of gasoline, the engine is probably flooded. Wait several minutes, then try again.

b. If your car's been sitting in the rain, wipe the spark plug wires with a dry rag. After about fifteen minutes it should be dry enough to start.

c. If the car is extremely cold, press the gas pedal to the floor two or three times and try starting. You may have to try several times, but wait awhile in between tries. If the engine shows no sign of life, stop trying before you run the battery down. If possible, call for a service truck. If not, you can remove the battery and take it inside. An hour or two of warmth will often allow battery power to build up enough to start your car.

d. If the battery is completely dead, you must have it recharged. To prepare for this emergency, keep a pair of jumper cables in your car. These cables transfer power from a "live" battery to a "dead" one.

To use jumper cables, position the car with a live battery nose to nose with the one with a dead battery. With the dead car turned off, attach the cables to the battery terminals of each car. The red goes to the positive post (+) and the black cable to the negative post (-). Race the engine of the car with the good battery. Depress the accelerator on the dead car once, then start the engine. Once the engine is running, release the black cables from both batteries, and then the red ones.

2. *Flat tires*

   a. Keep a jack and lug wrench in your car.

   b. Make sure the spare tire is properly inflated.

   c. If you have a flat, pull well off the road, have passengers get out and stand away from the car. Switch on your emergency flashers, turn off the engine, and apply the parking brake. If driving a stick shift, leave it in gear; if driving an automatic transmission, leave it in park.

   d. Remove the jack and spare tire from the trunk. Using the lug wrench, pry the hubcap off the wheel. Use the lug wrench to loosen the nuts, but don't remove them yet. (Usually the nuts must be turned counterclockwise.) Place the jack under the jacking point on the bumper. (The Owner's Manual will tell you where that point is, or you may find instructions on a label affixed to the trunk.) Make sure the base of the jack is set firmly on the ground and jack up the car until the wheel is barely off the ground.

   e. Making sure that the car is stable on the jack (try rocking the car a time or two; it should be stable), remove the lug nuts. Lift the wheel off and put the spare on. Tighten the lug nuts back onto the wheel so that they are finger-tight. Lower the car until the new tire is resting on the ground but not carrying the full weight of the car. Then tighten the nuts with the lug wrench and lower the car completely. Tighten the lug nuts again as firmly as possible.

   f. Stop at the next service station and make sure everything is o.k.

3. Running out of gas

If you should run out of gas, the symptoms will be a smoothly running car which suddenly begins to hesitate, come to life again, and cough erratically. If this happens, pull off the road immediately. Turn on your emergency flashers, check the fuel gauge to see if it's on empty; flick it with your finger to see if it's stuck. If it doesn't read empty, remove the gas tank cap and rock the car. You'll be able to hear gasoline sloshing if there's any in the tank.

If the tank is empty, lock your car, leaving the emergency flashers on. If you're on a limited-access highway, stay off the road and wait for help from a state highway patrolman. (Remember that "Please Call Police" sign you carry for emergencies?) On other roads, you may—if you're a man—choose to walk to the nearest telephone or service station. Since many stations don't have gasoline cans for such emergencies, it's best to keep an empty can and a funnel with a flexible spout in the trunk of your car. A gallon of gas will usually get you to a service station.

When you get back to the car with the gas, pour all but a capful of gas into the tank and try to start the engine. You may have to let it turn over several times, but wait in between times. If the battery seems to be weak, stop this procedure; you'll have to prime the carburetor. Lift the hood and remove the wing nut attaching a disk-like lid which is the air cleaner. Pour about a quarter of the remaining gasoline into the carburetor opening, replace the air cleaner and try to start the engine. You may have to prime the carburetor several times. If there is gas in the car and the weather is very cold, your fuel line may be frozen. The solution for that problem is to get your car into a heated place until the line thaws. You can also buy gas line anti-freeze (dry gas) and pour it into the tank to avoid future freezing.

4. Radiator boils over

Watch the temperature gauge and try to stop the car and pull off the road when the light signals overheating.

Turn off the air conditioner. Put the car into neutral and

race the engine. When you pull off the road, turn off the engine, raise the hood, and give the car at least thirty minutes to cool off.

Proper maintenance should enable you to avoid most emergency situations.

In recent months we've seen a lot of older cars on the road. Dealers vie with each other, constantly advertising all kinds of "super" deals and low interest rates on their latest models. Yet new car sales are down.

"I haven't bought a new car in twenty years," said one whose financial expertise I highly respect. I notice he does a lot of flying. He drives on short trips only.

"If you really take care of a car," another financial counselor said, "you should be able to drive it 150,000 miles."

His wife's car has 98,000 on it. She suggested we trade ours—with 24,000—in on a new one. She'd like to buy ours.

In spite of the experts' advice, I have an attack of car fever every two years. There's only one known cure for that.

My husband has more resistance to it than I have. In fact, when I take the car in for service, he practically forbids me to step inside the showroom. He knows it's dangerous for me to talk to a salesman. That is, unless the salesman's a chauvinist. I've met a few.

A few days after my cousin, Vera, married, she came back to her parents' home to clean out her desk and prepare to move her things. Watching every move Vera made, her three-year-old niece clattered constantly. My uncle came along just in time to see a stack of old letters hit the wastebasket.

"Vera, you ought to look through those letters. There might be some money in them," he cautioned.

"Money! Money!" snorted the child. "Dat's all he tink about!"

My uncle liked to tell that incident and laugh about it. He knew he had a reputation for craving money.

Naturally, we don't want to become overly concerned with material things. The Scripture warns us about that.

But money is all right as long as we use it wisely and don't let it control us.

Hopefully what we've learned from this visit to Commerce Drive will help us to better manage our financial affairs for the enrichment of our lives and the lives of our families.

Chapter 8
Crestview Development: Housing Facilities

Although many senior citizens own their homes and prefer to remain in them indefinitely, other people want to move. As we examine alternate housing arrangements, we'll stop at a real estate office for some suggestions.

Location

Unless you must move to a different area because of health problems, you can save yourself anxiety and money by investigating the location before you move. If possible, spend time there—during different seasons. The climate may be perfect in May but unbearable in August. Subscribe to the newspaper to learn more about the place. Get acquainted with people who live there.

If moving to another section of your city, consider the accessibility of your proposed new home to important places and people. You'll want to be near your doctor, grocery store, post office, church, public transportation, and, hopefully, family.

Check the area for safety. After showing several homes to a prospect, one real estate agent said of a house near the lake:

"I wouldn't recommend this house to you since your husband works out of town."

Not all realtors are that concerned with your safety. You'll probably have to find out from someone else.

Get acquainted with some of the neighbors. What are they like? Are they your kind of people? Do you "belong" there? Is the environment pleasant?

Answers to such questions should help you decide if you want to move there.

Type of Housing

If you own or rent a house, you may want to maintain it as long as possible. On the other hand, you may decide it's too big, too much work to keep up the lawn, too much expense for utilities and up-keep, too far from the children or other significant people and places. You may want a safer, smaller, less expensive home.

A condominium could be your answer. You will be living close to others. You will have little or no lawn. If you want less space, you can get it. You may even be able to arrange with a friend to buy an adjoining condominium. You'll probably have money left over from the sale of your house, if you have built up much equity in one. Selling a condominium can present problems, but maybe your heirs will have to deal with them.

If the condominium isn't for you, maybe you'd like an apartment. Less space, no yard, close neighbors, a maintenance person, a night watchman—many features entice senior adults to apartment complexes. Some drawbacks include untrustworthy maintenance help and fire hazard. With some of your own furniture, however, you can probably adjust to apartment living and learn to enjoy it.

Some older people buy or rent mobile homes. These can be located near the children perhaps. They provide inexpensive housing—compared to some other facilities. But major problems include temperature control, danger of severe weather, undesirable neighbors, and lack of safe environment.

Retirement communities are springing up all around the country. If you really prefer the company of your age group, the country-club atmosphere, the luxury of food, fun, freedom, investigate a retirement community. Notice I said, "Investigate." As with other housing choices, this one requires careful investigation. Keep your house, condo, or apartment long enough to try the village for 30 days. If you enjoy that style of living and can keep up the pace, you may decide to stay.

Similar to, yet different from, the retirement community is the life-care facility. Whereas the former is more like a village; the latter is more like an apartment complex with home-care facilities. As we become dependent, we may find this type of housing meets our needs better.

Home sharing is popular in different parts of the country. It may involve from two friends with similar tastes and interests to a dozen or so virtual strangers living in the same house as a family. Advantages of such an arrangement include companionship, cheaper housing, relative safety, and mutual caring. Disadvantages include personality conflicts, lack of privacy, and separation from natural families. Of course, with only a few friends sharing a home, the problems are minimal.

Selling Real Estate

Occasionally someone decides to sell a house without having to pay an agent's fee. "For Sale by Owner" signs in yards or in the Classified Ad column of a newspaper may bring results. But most people prefer to pay the extra fee for professional help. For them, trying to sell a house themselves isn't worth the hassle. And they have to pay someone to complete the transaction anyhow.

The real estate agent or broker is hired by you, the seller, to find a buyer for your property who will give you the best price. In return, you agree to pay him his fee once the deal is completed. No sale, no fee.

For this fee, he will screen prospective buyers, advertise, show your home by appointment, get the best price, and close the deal.

Buying a Home

Since buying your home is probably your largest single investment, and most homes for sale are listed with a realtor, you can take advantage of his services without additional cost.

Before buying our present home, I called a realtor and explained what we wanted. She selected twenty homes to show us. I'm sure she helped us get the best for our money.

Whatever type of housing you select, you and your family will probably be happier if you remain independent in your own living quarters as long as you possibly can.

If you can't live alone, try to get someone to stay with you. If that doesn't work, find a place that cares for older people.

If you must give up your home, do so temporarily. When a friend who lives alone scheduled surgery, she made arrangements to spend a month in a nursing home upon her release from the hospital. After that month, she went home. Some of us would have given up and moved into the nursing home.

Four years ago, Herbert, a friend in his 80's, fell off a ladder and hit his head on the driveway. Everyone thought he had a heart attack. His daughter came from out of state. As soon as he could leave the hospital, she put him in a nursing home. Later, he transferred to another nursing home. But he wasn't happy. When we visited him, he was depressed. Months later, he went home. He still lives alone and seems much more alert. He drives his car to church almost every Sunday.

Of course if we live alone, we run the risk of dying alone. But maybe it's worth the risk.

I used to say that to my mother when she chose to live alone. She died in her 85th year after seven weeks in a nursing home and seven in the hospital. As traumatic as her dying alone would have been, I wish she had slipped away to be with her Lord in the privacy of her own home. She would have preferred that way too.

If you live alone, start a telephone reassurance program. Enlist a number of friends. Each person calls certain ones every morning to see if they are all right. Thus, the caller has a responsibility and the person called has a feeling of security. The caller can report illnesses or accidents to family members of the one called. Possibilities of this program are unlimited. It can become a channel for news, information, or just a chance to talk.

Consider moving in with your children only as a last resort. Be sure you've explored all other options. Even then, keep your home, condo, apartment, or whatever for a month at least. Move in on a trial basis only. Test the arrangement to see if it will work. It seldom does.

After a few weeks, you may recover from whatever illness or condition that prompted the move. Your son or daughter may feel torn between you and a spouse and children. His or her spouse may resent your intrusion into their home. The children may be disrespectful, noisy, and intolerant.

Their music may drive you up the wall. But if you have no place to go home to, you're forced to suffer in silence or cause trouble for those you love.

Ten years ago at age 85, Tom had one kidney removed. No one expected him to live. From the hospital, he went to a nursing home for a few weeks. Meanwhile, Anna stayed with their son Carl and his wife Sue and three teenage children.

Months later, Tom left the hospital. They sold their home and furniture. Carl and Sue took them in. Anna complained constantly about the situation, especially about the teenagers—their dress, their music, their friends.

After Tom's health improved, he and Anna could have stayed in their home had they not sold it. They could have rented an apartment and lived alone. But they didn't. At last the time came that they couldn't care for themselves. The teenagers married and left home. Sue continued to care for Tom and Anna. Since Anna's death, Sue still cares for Tom, a remarkably active 95-year-old.

Commendable on Sue's part, but it has taken ten years of her life. Much of that time unnecessarily.

With the various aids available to the elderly, you should be able to remain independent indefinitely.

Community Services

A number of organizations work together to enable a

senior citizen to live alone. These services include the following:

1. Title III Meal Program
For those 60 and older, this program provides a low-cost or free meal in a congregate setting. This meal includes one-third of the Recommended Dietary Allowance. Transportation, information regarding other services, health counseling, nutrition education, and recreational activities are a part of the program.

2. Meals on Wheels
Civic clubs, hospitals, and other groups sponsor the meals on wheels program. They deliver to the home one hot, well balanced meal daily (except weekends), for a minimal charge. The cost is usually based on the recipient's ability to pay.

3. Day-Care Program
This is a health care institution or a Senior Citizen's center. The elderly can stay there during the day, using their own abilities to help others and sharing experiences, talents, knowledge, skills, and themselves.

A pleasant, safe environment, immediate access to skilled medical attention, self-care training—including dressing and grooming—group leisure-time activities, supervised administration of required medication, and at least one nutritious meal a day make Day-Care and Senior Citizens' centers very popular among older adults.

4. Adult Foster Care Program
This program provides short-term or long-term help for the elderly.

Our neighbor and her husband recently brought her 95-year-old grandmother to live with them. The couple takes turns working at the same job. They made arrangements for a sitting service to relieve them occasionally. One such service advertises staff members available on a 24-hour basis in the event of an emergency. They prepare meals, follow a medication schedule, and help the old person to dress, exercise, and bathe. The cost of such services, according to the advertisement, is $6.35 per hour, with a minimum of three hours' service.

In many cases government funds are available for companions, legal and tax advice, and transportation.

The following home safety tips should prove helpful:

Rugs, Runners, and Mats

1. Remove rugs and runners that tend to slide.
2. Apply double-faced adhesive carpet tape or rubber.
3. Buy rugs with slip-resistant backing.
4. Check periodically to see if backing should be replaced.
5. Place rubber matting under rugs. (It can be cut to size.)

Telephone Area

1. Keep near the telephone numbers for the Police, Fire Department, Ambulance, Poison Control Center, and a neighbor.
2. Write the above numbers in large print and tape them to or near the phone.
3. Have at least one telephone located where it would be accessible in the event of an accident which leaves you unable to stand.

Smoke Detectors

1. Buy at least one smoke detector for each floor of your home.
2. Follow the instructions that come with the smoke detector concerning the best place to install it.
3. Place the detector near bedrooms, either on the ceiling or 6-12 inches below the ceiling on the wall.
4. Locate smoke detectors away from air vents.
5. Check and replace batteries and bulbs according to the manufacturer's instructions.
6. Vacuum the grillwork of your detector.

Electrical Outlets and Switches

1. Check for warm or hot outlets or switches that may indicate an unsafe wiring condition.
2. Unplug cords from outlets and do not use the switches if they're hot.
3. Have an electrician check the wiring immediately.
4. Exposed wiring presents a shock hazard. Add a cover plate.

Light Bulbs

Use a bulb of the correct type and wattage. (If you do not know the correct wattage, use a bulb no larger than 60 watts.) Ceiling fixtures, recessed lights, and "hooded" lamps will trap heat.

Space Heaters

1. Never defeat the grounding feature provided by a 3-hole receptacle or an adapter for a 2-hole receptacle designed to lessen the risk of shock.
2. If you do not have a 3-hole outlet, use an adapter to connect the heater's 3-prong plug.
3. Make sure the adapter ground wire or tab is attached to the outlet.
4. Relocate heaters away from passageways and flammable materials such as curtains, rugs, furniture, etc.
5. Unvented heaters should be used with room doors open or window slightly open to provide ventilation. The correct fuel, as recommended by the manufacturer, should always be used. Vented heaters should have proper venting, and the venting system should be checked frequently. This is the most frequent cause of carbon monoxide poisoning, and older people are at special risk.
6. Follow installation and operating instructions.
7. Call your fire department if you have further questions.

Woodburning Heating Equipment

1. Get a qualified person to install woodburning stoves according to local building codes.
2. Call local building code officials or the fire marshall for requirements and recommendations for installation.

   Note: Some insurance companies will not cover fire losses if wood stoves are not installed according to local codes.

Emergency Exit Plan

1. Develop an emergency exit plan.
2. Choose a meeting place outside your home so you can be sure that everyone has escaped.
3. Practice the plan occasionally to be sure everyone can escape quickly and safely.

Kitchen

I. Range Area
   A. Store flammable and combustible items away from the range and oven.
   B. Remove any towels hanging on oven handles. If towels hang close to a burner, change the location of the towel rack.
   C. If necessary, shorten or remove curtains that could brush against heat sources.
   D. Roll back long, loose sleeves or fasten them with pins or elastic bands while you are cooking.
   E. Use ventilation systems or open windows to clear the air of vapors and smoke.

II. Electrical Cords
   A. Move cords and appliances away from sink areas and hot surfaces.
   B. Move appliances closer to wall outlets or to different outlets so you won't need extension cords.
   C. If extension cords must be used, install wiring

guides so that cords will not hang near the sink, range, or working areas.
D. Consider adding new outlets for convenience and safety. Install outlets equipped with *ground fault circuit interrupters* (GFCIs) to protect against electric shock. A GFCI is a shock-protection device that will detect electrical fault and shut off electricity before serious injury or death occurs.

III. Lighting
A. Open curtains and blinds.
B. Use the maximum wattage bulb allowed by the fixture. (If you don't know, use a bulb no larger than 60 watts.)
C. Reduce glare by using frosted bulbs, indirect lighting, shades or globes on light fixtures, or partially closing blinds or curtains.
D. If necessary, install additional light fixtures.
E. Look for safety warnings on bulb size on lamps and fixtures.

IV. Step Stool
A. If you don't own a step stool, buy one.
B. Choose one with a handrail you can hold onto while standing on the top step.
C. Before climbing on a step stool, make sure it is fully opened and stable.
D. Tighten screws and braces on the step stool.
E. Discard those with broken parts.

Living Room/Family Room

I. Rugs and Runners—check them.
II. Electrical and Telephone Cords
A. Make sure cords are not frayed.
B. Keep cords out of traffic where they can trip you.
C. Don't let furniture rest on cords.
III. Fireplace and Chimney
A. Do not use a clogged chimney.
B. Have the chimney checked and cleaned by a regis-

tered or licensed professional.
IV. Passageways
A. Install night lights.
B. Avoid tripping hazards.

Bathroom
I. Bathtub and Shower Areas
A. Apply textured strips or appliques on the floors of tubs and showers.
B. Use non-skid mats in the tub or shower and on the bathroom floor.
C. If you are unsteady on your feet, use a stool with non-skid tips as a seat while showering or bathing.
D. Attach grab bars to structural supports in the wall, or install specifically designed bars that attach to the sides of the bathtub.

II. Water Temperature
A. Lower the setting on your hot water heater to "Low" or 120 degrees.
B. Always check water temperature by hand before entering bath or shower.
C. Taking baths, rather than showers, reduces the risk of a scald from suddenly changing water temperatures.

III. Lighting
A. Install a light switch near the door.
B. Install a night light.
C. Replace the existing switch with a "glow switch" that can be seen in the dark.

IV. Small Electrical Appliances
A. Unplug small appliances when they're not in use.
B. Never reach into water to retrieve an appliance without being sure the appliance is unplugged.

V. Medications
A. Be sure all containers are clearly marked with the contents, doctor's instructions, expiration date, and patient's name.

B. Dispose of outdated medicines properly.
C. Request non-child-resistant closures from your pharmacist only when you're sure no children will be in your home.

Bedrooms

I. Areas Around Beds
A. Place furniture near lamps or switches.
B. Install night lights.
C. Remove sources of heat or flame from areas around beds.
D. Don't smoke in bed.
E. Use electric blankets according to the manufacturer's instructions.
F. Don't allow anything, including other blankets or comforters or pets, on top of the electric blanket while it is in use.
G. Don't set an electric blanket so high that it could burn someone who falls asleep while it is on.
H. Avoid tucking in the sides or ends of your electric blanket.
I. Never go to sleep with a heating pad on, even on a low setting.

II. Telephone
Place a telephone within reach of your bed.

Stairs

I. Lighting
A. Locate a switch at the top and bottom.
B. Install night lights.
C. Keep a flashlight handy.

II. Handrails
Install handrails on both sides of the stairway and the total length of the stairway.

Once you've found whatever housing arrangement best fits your needs, following the above suggestions should help you avoid accidents and tragedies.

Chapter 9
Bel-Aire Circle: Physical Health Facilities

We're now entering the medical complex called Bel-Aire Circle. As we enjoy a balanced meal in the hospital cafeteria, a dietician will explain special nutritional needs of older people. After lunch, a doctor from the adjoining clinic will tell us about the physical side of the aging process. We'll also visit the gym to learn about exercise appropriate for us. Finally, we'll stop by the nursing home, where five percent of the elderly live. This medical complex offers hope for our citizens to live and die with dignity.

Compared to physical health, all other blessings fade into insignificance. A child stricken with a serious illness, an adolescent forced to surrender dreams and ambitions for an invalid's existence, a young parent struggling with a life-threatening disease that will disrupt the entire family, or a grandparent in the throes of pain—all provoke our sympathy. We delve into our pockets for whatever is necessary, even costly, experimental organ transplants. To most of us, life and health have no price tags.

As we age, however, we expect to have health problems, to "wear out" gradually. Modern medicine enables us to postpone, and in some cases to prevent, many health hazards if we take necessary precautions. "A healthy diet, sensible exercise, and avoidance of excessive drug intake are some of the key factors in helping the middle-aged adult remain healthy."[1] If we have ignored these key factors in middle age, we may still be able to reap benefits by giving attention to them regardless of our age.

Nutrition

We don't like to be reminded that we are what we eat.

When anyone suggests a change in our dietary habits, we say, "You can't teach an old dog new tricks." We would punch someone in the nose if he called us an old dog. Yet we rely comfortably on the old cliche to justify our behavior. Since we aren't dogs, we can learn new behavior patterns—including a change in our diets.

After losing some weight at my doctor's insistence, I complained about my wrinkles. He snapped, "You may be around longer to have more wrinkles." Who knows? He's probably right. Obesity can raise blood cholesterol, blood pressure, and blood sugar in some patients. But obesity is not the only nutritional concern.

In "Dietary Needs in Later Life," Nell Robinson gives the following suggestions for menu planning:
1. Serve meals on a regular schedule.
2. Include a variety.
3. Eat smaller amounts more often.
4. Consider food a good investment.
5. Be aware of food and drug interaction.
6. Prepare and serve food attractively.
7. Drink lots of water.
8. Eat foods high in fiber.
9. Season food to make it taste good.
10. Use polyunsaturated oils and margarines.
11. Use meat substitutes—cheese, dried beans, and peanut butter.
12. Eat fresh fruits and vegetables.
13. Eat whole grain or enriched breads and cereals.[2]

A decreasing sensitivity of taste buds in older people can cause under-nutrition that leads to serious problems.[3] To compensate for taste sensitivity, we may use too much salt. Salt, in turn, can cause water retention and elevate blood pressure. My doctor says it can take up to two weeks to get rid of the salt in one meal. Restaurant food tends to be too salty. Only recently some cafeteria chains are advertising less salty food. Hopefully, others will follow suit.

Not only can too much salt cause problems, but doctors concerned with high levels of cholesterol warn against eating too many eggs. Some say we may safely eat two or three eggs per week; others suggest we not eat eggs, especially the yolks.

In addition to eggs, which tend to elevate cholesterol levels, fat must be rationed. "Most physicians and nutritionists," says Peggy Kloster Yen, "agree that it is wise for older adults to eat less fat."[4] We do need some fat. Yen recommends no more than 30 to 35 percent of calories in the older person's diet be from fats.[5] Too much can raise cholesterol levels.

In Lipid Research Clinics studies, reducing blood cholesterol levels by 10 percent decreased incidents of heart disease in participants by some 20 percent.[6]

Yen concludes:

"Although most of us can reduce our blood cholesterol by changes in diet, age itself is the most potent risk factor for heart disease. The older a person, the more likely a heart attack or stroke. But while aging cannot be halted, diet can be modified."[7]

Not only is a high fat diet likely to increase our risk of heart disease, but it may also be a factor in colon and breast cancer. "Because this is a long-term effect, however, it is difficult to know whether a dietary change in late life will be beneficial."[8]

Including fiber in our diet tends to reduce the risk of colon cancer. The second most common cancer in men, the third most common in women, colon-rectal cancer attacked 126,000 and took the lives of 58,100 in 1983.[9] Although prognosis in early detection is good, prevention is far better. If eating more fiber helps, then fiber belongs in our diet.

What can and should we eat to maintain good health? Weight Watchers International recommends the following minimum daily servings of each of six categories of food:

	For Women	For Men
Fruit	3	4-6
Vegetables	2 (½ cup)	2 (½ cup)
Milk (low-fat)	2 (8 oz.)	2 (8 oz.)
Bread	2-3 (1 sl.)	4-5 (1 sl.)
Fat	3 (1 tsp.)	3 (1 tsp.)
Protein	6-8 (1 oz.)	8-10 (1 oz.)[10]

(Numbers in parentheses indicate one-serving amounts.)

The President's Task Force on Aging (1970) determined the major causes of malnutrition among older Americans as follows:

1. Insufficient income
2. Loneliness
3. Going to store too great a burden
4. Nutritional ignorance
5. Inability to prepare a hot meal.[11]

Various service clubs and other organizatoins are trying to help meet the nutritional needs of the elderly. A later chapter will discuss these projects along with other resources available to older people.

Exercise

No matter where we look we see physical fitness fanatics. On the basketball court or football field, at school, on the tennis court or hiking trail in the park, on the street in front of our homes, people of all ages play, run, jog, or walk. Sometimes it makes us tired just to watch them. We may envy their energy and enthusiasm. Or we may turn away in disgust and settle back in our recliner.

If you have lived a sedentary life, you could not, even if you dared try, jog three miles tomorrow. In fact, no one suggests strenuous exercise for an elderly person unless that activity is habitual. On the other hand, medical authorities agree that we do need exercise. Our own doctor can tell us what and how much.

Many of us ignore all efforts to get us out of our easy

chairs, sometimes even out of bed. After punching a clock for years, we deserve this promised leisure. It's easy to sleep in or spend hours sitting around reading the paper after breakfast. If that's what you really want, you'll probably get plenty of it. Soon you may not be able to do anything else.

If you don't want to exercise, you can always find an excuse. You don't need it. It's too risky. You mow the lawn every week. You're too old. You don't have time.

For those who refuse to atrophy, a regular, sensible exercise program can add zest and years to life. It may help avoid heart disease, joint and muscle problems, and stress-related illnesses.

Before launching an exercise program, however, you will be wise to consult your doctor. Unless you are in fairly good condition already, the doctor will likely recommend something mild or moderate that you can work up to gradually.

Walking ranks high among the exercises recommended. In his article "Talking About Walking," Bill Gale says, "Medical doctors coast to coast, along with the American Heart Association, recommend this muscle-stretching, cardiovascular-stimulating exercise as the very best way to keep fit for anyone, at any age." Gale advocates walking as a safe, free, available-all-day exercise that makes one look and feel good. He recommends it for additional reasons:

1. Muscles stretch,
2. Shed pounds,
3. Keep in shape,
4. Fun,
5. Relieves stress and anxiety,
6. Nurtures and refreshes body, mind, and spirit,
7. Safe,
8. Natural,
9. Companionable,
10. No competition.[12]

Most of us have an area for walking within reach of our

homes. If we can't walk in our own neighborhood, we can drive to a nearby park. Shopping malls provide space for walking. Unpleasant weather is no excuse. If confined inside, we can walk for 20 to 30 minutes in the house.

Walk 2 or 3 blocks to the next bus stop, park your car a few blocks from your destination, climb a flight or two of stairs instead of taking the elevator. Start anywhere.

Stress Reducing Tips

1. Get to know your body. Shallow breathing and frequent fast pulse are an indication of your body's reaction to stress.
2. Learn to relax. Deep breathing is a NATURAL RELAXANT. Try to take several deep breaths every hour.
3. Practice this simple exercise to help you relax: Tense all your muscles, hold for a count of five, then let go. Do this five times a day and notice the difference.
4. At the end of the day, take a brisk walk, do a few minutes of fast dancing or body shaking. This stimulating exercise will loosen you up and get your blood flowing.
5. Smile—you will be surprised how good it makes you and others feel.
6. Practice unwinding every day. Don't wait for your annual vacation. Your body is the only one you'll get down here, so be good to it!
7. Have fun. Learn to play a little. Plan frequent mini-trips and outings. Sometimes, all it takes is some creative thinking.
8. Take a walk at lunchtime. Get out of the office or house. Fresh air clears the brain, and the change of scenery helps you to relax.
9. Be aware of your frequent need for relaxation times in your day. Try this simple exercise: Stand up and stretch like a cat, then close your eyes for five min-

utes and pretend you're walking on the beach or fishing in a cool brook. Teach yourself to relax.
10. Limit your intake of caffeinated beverages.
11. Begin your day with some limbering up and simple stretching exercises, then jog in place for a few minutes. This routine will help you warm up and get started for the day.
12. Keeping fit helps prevent stress problems. Vigorous exercise is a great way to get rid of the uptight stressed feeling.
13. Take your aggressions out on the tennis court, golf course, swimming pool, etc.
14. Learn to make lists.
15. Take control of your own life.[13]

Dr. Robert N. Butler says that if exercise could be put in a pill, it would be the most prescribed and the most beneficial medicine in the country.

Let's try it and walk to the clinic.

Aging, meet Mankind; Mankind, this is Aging.

Aging: I have known you for sometime but I doubt you recognize me.
Mankind: Oh! and how is that?
Aging: It is my policy not to force myself upon one until I've known that person for some years.
Mankind: I'm shocked. Have you known me that long?
Aging: Well, yes. I left my card but you never read it. It is with you still but then like most, you won't acknowledge it until—
Mankind: Really? Where?
Aging: Your arteries, my friend![14]

King Solomon paints a vivid picture of old age: Failing eyesight, trembling hands, feeble knees, decaying teeth, deafness, insomnia, lagging interest, fear, weakness, lack of sexual desire, kidney and heart failure—all are included in his image (Eccl. 12:1-7).

With the help of medical doctors, we can compile a similar list of common physical changes in the elderly:

I. *Skin*—Wrinkles, rough surface, and spots of dark pigment appear. The skin becomes more vulnerable to cancer, loss of hair, bruises, and dryness. But it is still able to protect beyond 120 years.

II. *Stiff Joints*—Hips and knees especially become stiff, causing a bent posture.

III. *Muscles*—After age 70, loss of muscular strength is evident.

IV. *Menopause*—Women usually feel better afterward.

V. *Nervous System*—Hardening of the arteries causes circulatory problems in the brain and reduced speed for processing information and sending signals for action. Most of us begin to notice these changes in the late 40's. And failure of the circulatory system is the most common cause of death in people over age 40.

Problems with the nervous system affect perception. Reaction time increases. Speed of movement declines. And processing of stimuli takes more time. The patient tends to underestimate the passage of time, to be less capable of judging the speed of a moving object, and to be more cautious and indecisive.

VI. *Kidneys and Bladder*
   A. Kidneys perform only half as well in a person over 80 as in one in the 20's.
      1. It takes longer to concentrate waste products into urine.
      2. The kidneys are not so effective in retaining a balance of fluids.
   B. Bladder capacity decreases.
      1. There is less awareness of the need to urinate until the bladder is almost full.
      2. As a result, the patient suffers kidney and bladder infections.

VII. *Sensory Changes*
   A. Vision
      1. Ability to focus on near objects decreases.

    2. Lens and iris show decline.
    3. Distinguishing levels of brightness becomes difficult.
    4. Twenty-five percent of those over 70 have cataracts.
    5. Only a small percent of people are blind, but blindness is more common among the elderly.
    6. Failing eyesight is often the first noticeable change.
B. Hearing
    1. It is difficult for the elderly to hear high-pitched or low intensity sounds. Older people can more easily hear voices, horns, telephones, and doorbells with a low tone and high intensity.
    2. Impaired hearing reduces capacity for interaction with others. It often causes embarrassment and misunderstanding.

"Martha," the old gentleman began, as the two relaxed after celebrating their Golden Wedding Anniversary, "I'm proud of you."

"Well, that's all right," came the terse reply, "I'm tired of you too."

No wonder no other change in later life has a more dramatic effect on its victim.

The most prominent effect is a sense of anxiety and, in many cases, serious depression. It can arouse suspicion when its victim has trouble understanding what family members and others are saying.

Family members become reluctant to repeat everything they say.

This situation may lead to paranoia in the hearing impaired person.

Sometimes medical treatment will help. Often a hearing aid will improve one's hearing dramatically. But this is a very sensitive subject. It's strange that elderly people will readily agree to wearing eyeglasses or dentures or walking with a cane. But they will stubbornly refuse to accept a hearing aid.

If your physician recommends a hearing aid, why not try and judge for yourself whether it helps? It may take some getting used to, but if you need one, it may well be worth the cost and inconvenience. As for its appearance, it is scarcely noticeable—certainly not as much as your hearing impairment.

VIII. *Respiration*—Increased breathing difficulties are probably caused by "a decreased absorption surface within the lungs and a reduction in their capacity for elastic recoil." This condition threatens the survival of cells, especially in the brain, which needs oxygen. Depriving the brain of sufficient oxygen causes confusion, disorientation, and if prolonged, structural brain damage, resulting in mental deterioration, lack of coordination, and death. Contrary to common belief, this condition is not senility.[15]

IX. *Cardiovascular System*—Arteries become narrower, less flexible, and plugged up. Arteriosclerosis is like a water pipe in which rust has built up over the years. The more corroded the pipe or the artery, the greater the risk of rupture when water or blood is forced against the obstruction. This condition in the arteries causes high blood pressure, because the heart must work harder to force the blood through. And it sets the stage for death by heart attack, kidney failure, or stroke.

As arteries harden, according to one doctor, a person automatically becomes either very bitter or very sweet.

X. *Bones*—Especially common in women after menopause, *osteoporosis* —thinning of the bone—affects to some degree all aging persons. Osteoporosis is a major cause of hip, wrist, or spine fractures; back pain; and the so-called dowager's hump.

We often hear that some elderly person fell and broke a hip. Probably the truth is that he or she broke a hip, then fell.

The best way to prevent osteoporosis is moderate exercise, an estrogen supplement for post-menopausal women, and a calcium-rich diet. Adults need 1,000 to 1,500 milligrams of calcium daily. The best source of calcium is dairy products. One cup of whole milk, for example, contains almost 300 milligrams of calcium.

Other calcium-rich foods include the following:
1. Sardines, salmon, shrimp, and oysters
2. Collard greens, kale, broccoli, and bean curd
3. Yogurt
4. Ice cream
5. Cheese

According to Dr. Richard Rivlin, nutritional specialist, calcium deficiency may contribute to high blood pressure and colon cancer as well as to osteoporosis. He recommends 800 to 1,000 milligrams per day. To get that amount of calcium, he suggests foods such as meat, vegetables, cereals, and fruits, in addition to dairy products.

Dr. Rivlin warns that one can get too much calcium. In susceptible people, too much may cause kidney stones.[16]

XI. *Digestive System*

Problems in the digestive system are more likely the result of poor eating and drinking habits than of aging.

Preventive Health Care

Preventive health care measures include the following:
1. Periodic physical examination
2. Accident prevention
3. Good nutrition
4. Exercise

"Rapidity of aging depends on a person's heredity, lifelong dietary patterns, the amount of habitual exercise, past illnesses, the presence of one or more chronic illnesses, and the stresses experienced throughout life."[17]

"We used to assume," says Dr. Illene Siegler, chief psychologist in a long-term study at Duke University, "that later life was a period of decline, without excitement. Now we know that physical health variables are what you should worry about and not age itself."[18]

"Because some consider mental decline a natural part of aging, they may ignore symptoms that really derive from treatable physical disease or from reversible depression."[19] Forgetfulness isn't a "normal" part of aging. The fact that a person can't remember recent events is usually a physical problem.

We now know that many symptoms formerly called senility are in fact a disease. Alzheimer's disease strikes 5 to 10 percent of Americans over 65. But it is not a natural effect of aging. It can hit people as early as the 20's or 30's. One-half to three-fourths of all those people in nursing homes are victims of Alzheimer's.

The fourth leading killer in America, the disease affects 1.5 million Americans. Not enough research has been done to know much about preventing or treating the disease. Unfortunately, we do know something of its symptoms and results.

Since you have a 90 to 95 percent chance of not becoming a victim of Alzheimer's, your *senility* may very well be treatable.

For example, John's thinking was so slow that his family and friends said he was "senile." He could think clearly, but extremely slow. His doctor found out he needed a pace-maker. After receiving his pace-maker, John discovered his thinking had improved significantly.

Eighty-six percent of people over 65 have some chronic health problem for which they take medication. Eighty-four percent, however, are functionally healthy. John Chancellor reports that 75 percent of men aged 75 and up are in good health. "To stay young," Chancellor suggests, "be engaged in something you like to do."[20]

"When played with skill, the part of Old Person is marked by tranquility, wisdom, freedom, dignity, and a sense of humor. Almost everyone would like to play it that way, but few have the courage to try."[21]

Let's adopt George Burns' philosophy on aging: "Once you've lived to 100 you've really got it made because very few people die over 100."

We know that positive thinking helps us avoid heart attacks and strokes. But with cancer, our number two killer, shouldn't we ask if our emotions have anything to do with it?

Dr. Robert W. Bermudes thinks so. In his book *Conqering Cancer*, he cites a number of studies to support his claim.

"The lack of agreement in medical circles over the cause and cure of cancer," states Bermudes, "raises the possibility that what a person holds as 'truth' or important—one's belief system—is connected to some degree with that person's susceptibility to cancer."[22]

From various studies, Bermudes concludes that there is a cancer-prone personality. Characteristics of this personality include "grasping for control, possessive and manipulative" attitudes toward others, a "workaholic" disposition, with a sense of "hopelessness."

According to Bermudes, cancer diagnosis often follows within six months such traumatic events as the death of a loved one, divorce, retirement, or severe illness in the family.[23]

Other studies indicate that the passive person may be more susceptible to cancer. Often this individual has either lost a parent or been physically or emotionally distant from a parent during childhood. Consequently, he or she learns to repress emotions and may experience difficulty in forming and sustaining relationships.

Much cancer research suggests that small cancers form in all of us, but our immune system fights them off. Dr. Joan Borysenko, an instructor at Harvard Medical School, believes that a person's inability to cope with stress may weaken the immune system and impair its ability to combat disease. She contends that after the loss of a loved one or a valued job, the immune system may be especially weak and vulnerable. But she cautions against oversimplifying the relationships between stress, the immune system, and cancer.

Dr. Bernard Fox, of the National Cancer Institute, believes, however, that if indeed emotions affect the onset of cancer, they are only one of many factors.

Once cancer has been diagnosed, strong evidence indicates that victims with a fighting spirit are more successful than their passive counterparts in combating the disease.

According to a study of Englishwomen who had mastectomies for early-stage breast cancer:

women who reacted to the disease with a fighting spirit or strong denial were more likely to be cancer-free five years later than women who reacted with stoic acceptance or with feelings of hopelessness or helplessness. Women who felt they had control over the cancer had a better outlook than women who didn't.[24]

Whether attitudes can actually cause or prevent cancer may be debatable. But few would disagree that emotions can either facilitate or hinder the growth of malignant cells.

In addition to the major killers, a host of disabling or merely disagreeable physical ailments result from emotional turmoil. The Old Testament saint, Job, expressed a universal truth when he said, "For the thing which I greatly feared is come upon me, and that which I was afraid of is come unto me" (Job 3:25). And fear is only one emotion that causes problems. How we handle these destructive emotions determines the amount of gold or gloom in retirement.

With crime, natural disasters, and war portrayed constantly through the news media, we can hardly escape attacks of fear. In fact, world events divide us into three classes: (1) the fearful, (2) the faithful, (3) the uninformed. And often we fluctuate among the three.

The Nursing Home

More dreaded than heart attack, stroke, cancer, or death itself, the nursing home probably heads the list of fears among the elderly.

Lest you start dragging your feet as we approach this site, however, you may welcome some reassuring statistics: Only 5% of all those over age 65 live here. Of that number, 50 to 75% have Alzheimer's disease. Thus, you have a 95% chance of avoiding the nursing home. Very good odds, wouldn't you agree?

As they approached the mid-eighties, Mother and two other widows living next door to each other watched as their health slowly declined. Each struggled to remain independent in her own place as long as possible.

"I don't want you to break yourself down taking care of me," Mother used to say. "When I get to where I can't take care of myself, put me in a nursing home. I won't know much about it by that time anyhow."

Only one of those three ladies died in a nursing home. Mother spent a few weeks there, but she and the other lady went from their homes to the hospital where they died.

In that case, the odds were two to one against long-term nursing home residence.

Mother's statement, "I won't know much about it by that time anyhow," helps explain away some of my anxiety. What looks hopelessly depressing to me at 60 or 65 may not look nearly so bad at 85 or 90, when I can no longer take care of myself.

In one of my anxious moments, before I learned of my odds and thought of the difference in attitudes as we age, I seemed to hear the Lord's reassuring words: "If you ever have to go to a nursing home, I'll go with you." He didn't speak audibly, of course, but I believe He put the thought into my mind. It bears out the promise, "Lo, I am with you alway, *even* unto the end of the world" (Matt. 28:20).

When we visited Uncle Harvey in a nursing home last year, he seemed quite content. After his wife died, he lived alone until he was in his 90's. Once when we went by to see him, he had been shoveling snow off his driveway so he could drive to church. He was then 91. But eventually he decided he couldn't keep house and live alone any longer. He agreed that the children should put him in a nursing home. One day they took him back home. He walked around through the house and lay down a while. Then, he said, "It's time to go now." Later, he suggested that the children sell his house. He knew he could never live there alone again. A few weeks ago he died in the nursing home.

Edna has Alzheimer's disease. For years she could not get along with her son and family. She pestered anyone who would listen about imaginary problems—theft of items from her home, a neighbor breaking into her home at night, someone trying to get her money.

Police, lawyers, and bankers ignored her—at least as much as possible—when they discovered she was paranoid.

After offering to sell her home at a third of its value, she finally sold it far too cheap. Then she had her furniture moved over 400 miles three times before admitting she couldn't live alone.

Now she plays games with friends in the nursing home. When her family visits, she introduces them to her friends. She no longer spends a fortune on long-distance telephone calls for she's no longer lonely and scared.

Mary celebrated her 90th birthday recently. With her son and family, she enjoys church activities. She attends all the services of her church. And she plays the piano for some of the nursing home services; this despite the silicone joints that enable her to move fingers and toes. When she began losing her eyesight, she taught herself Braille. And she taught herself to type.

She asks everyone who visits her to read to her. She is still vitally interested in learning.

We'll have to move right along, or she'll want you to read for her.

As we continue our rounds of the home, I'll mention several of its important features.

1. For one thing, it has an excellent reputation. It is highly recommended by the Better Business Bureau, State Department of Human Services' Aging division, and various social services personnel.

2. The rooms are clean and odor-free. They have adequate space and lighting.

3. This home offers three levels of care: one for residents who can't take care of themselves, one for people with broken bones or short-term care problems, and one for residents who can take care of themselves but need

supervision.

4. It provides separate dining rooms for different kinds of residents. The food looks appetizing. And the kitchen facilities look immaculate.

5. The home accepts Medicare and Medicaid patients.

6. Admissions personnel screen roommates for compatibility.

7. There's a registered nurse on duty 24-hours a day.

8. For a minimal fee, the home provides transportation for patients to and from doctor's appointments.

9. It offers laundry services at no extra cost.

10. It has a beauty shop for the convenience of patients.

11. The home meets fire and safety standards.

12. A resident may have a television and a telephone, at his or her own expense.

In spite of all the plus factors of a nursing home, like any other move, it's wise to investigate before making irreversible decisions. A trial period, if feasible, is an excellent idea.

Carol lives alone. When she learned she would need surgery, she arranged with the nursing home to spend four weeks there upon dismissal from the hospital. With that decision behind her, Carol could focus on getting well. Her planning paid off.

In Carol's situation, however, many of us give up.

"I can't take care of myself after my operation," a less reasonable person would say. "I'll have to give up living alone and go to a nursing home."

Maybe so, for awhile. Not necessarily from now on.

Undoubtedly it takes courage to adjust to life in a nursing home. But if we're among the 5% who stay there—and among a lesser percent who realize what's going on—we will live one day at a time. Hopefully, we've already learned that lesson through God's Word. "Take therefore no thought for the morrow; for the morrow shall take thought for the things of itself," Jesus said. "Sufficient unto the day *is* the evil thereof" (Matt. 6:34).

Only a hypochondriac really enjoys a tour of a medical

complex. But we all like to know that when we or our loved one needs care, it is available. And Bel-Aire Circle medical complex offers hope for our citizens to live and die with dignity.

Age in Perspective

That stage of life you may in me behold
When all my aches and pain I so deplore
Remind me that this age is far from Gold
And make me long for joys I had before.

But as I turn the pages of the past
And flip from scene to scene of long ago,
I realize that though youth cannot last,
We need not think of Age as our fierce foe.

God did not plan for us to dwell on earth
Forever on this planet scarred by sin.
He figured from the moment of our birth,
We'd be worn out in threescore years and ten.

Old age is good when viewed in perspective,
Since we have only one alternative.

—Barkley

At our next stop, we concentrate on that alternative.
Though Sunset Parkway is beautiful, our stay here, for obvious reasons, will be brief.

Chapter 10
Sunset Parkway: Golden Acres Mortuary

The closer we come to this site, the slower our pace. Only severe physical or emotional pain entices one here. Even those of us who prepare for death itself often neglect to prepare for our funeral. But "as it is appointed unto men once to die" (Heb. 9:27), we might as well face the issue.

Pre-planning your funeral relieves survivors of the grueling task at a time of grief and probably exhaustion. It also assures you that your wishes will be carried out.

A few months before her death, Mother and I discussed her funeral arrangements. She told me which mortuary, cemetery, minister, singers, songs, and pallbearers she'd like to have.

Later, convinced that she would never leave the hospital alive, I met with the mortician and gave him the details. As a result, when Mother died, all I had to do was to call the funeral home. What a relief!

During my college days, a homiletics class scheduled a "funeral" at a local mortuary. A prankster in the class arranged to be placed in the casket before it was wheeled into the chapel. In the middle of the student preacher's sermon, the coffin lid opened slowly and the "corpse" sat up.

Despite jokes and crude attempts at humor—"Business is dead" or "I'm Digger O'Dell, your friendly undertaker. I'll be the last to let you down"—funerals aren't funny. Sometimes, however, they can be ironic.

For example, I sang for the funeral of a man who was buried in his wife's casket. Involved in an illicit love affair, he had bought a casket for his wife. By a twist of fate or act of God, he and the "other woman" died less than two weeks apart. The wife lived several years longer.

As we followed the hearse to the cemetery, I could almost see Haman swinging from the gallows he had prepared for Mordecai.

Let's get down to business now and see what's involved in pre-planning a funeral. I guarantee it will neither lengthen nor shorten your life.

Believe it or not, you're not required to have a funeral. You can opt for "direct disposition." In that event, your survivors need the services of a mortician to make sure they comply with state law.

For many reasons, most people prefer a funeral:

1. It provides meaningful ritual for individuals and close-knit groups.

2. It offers survivors social support—the presence of relatives and friends and other expressions of sympathy.

3. It helps survivors to adjust by forcing them to face reality. With a body present, one can't deny death. A mortician friend tells me that when a loved one's body is not recovered, survivors often experience extreme emotional problems.

4. It permits and encourages the bereaved to vent some of their deepest feelings of loss.

5. For many, it has a special religious meaning and value.

6. It is a means of giving testimony to a life that was lived.

7. It is a way of saying "goodbye" to that person who meant so much in a way that offers special meaning and appreciation.

Depending on where you live, you may have several possible choices for final disposition. Generally, your choices include the following:

1. Earth burial/Interment
2. Cremation
3. Entombment—mausoleum
4. Burial-at-Sea
5. Body donation

This choice is very important, because it is virtually irreversible.

Funeral expenses are generally determined by four factors:

1. Professional and staff services

These include removal of the body from the place of death, the care and preparation of the body, consultation with the family and clergy regarding the details for and conduct of the funeral or other post-death activity, preparation and filing of various legal documents and notices, and other assistance prior to, during, and following the funeral.

Care and preparation of the body generally includes embalming.

2. Facilities and equipment

This charge includes the use of funeral home facilities for the care and shelter of the body, the period of the wake or visitation, the funeral ceremony, plus the use of vehicles, equipment, and other facilities provided by the funeral home.

3. Merchandise

This includes the cost of the casket, the outer vault or liner (when earth burial is chosen), register books, memorial cards and in some instances, clothing.

4. Miscellaneous expenses

These may include paid newspaper notices, honoraria for clergy conducting the services, flowers, fees for musicians, and transportation of the body by common carrier, chartered aircraft, or casket coach if death occurs in a place other than where the funeral and disposition take place.

Costs vary according to the availability of the services and goods selected.

Some of the costs may be offset by various survivor's benefits, such as Social Security, Veterans Administration allowances, life insurance, Workmen's Compensation, union and fraternal organizations, burial societies, insurance coverage for accidental deaths, state veteran burial benefits, and state or local welfare allowances. Some states also provide benefits to those who survive the victim of a crime.

Your funeral director can explain these benefits and help determine whether your survivors qualify.

Prearranged funeral plans should allow for some flexibility. For example, when Mother died, her pastor was in Canada. We chose another staff member from her church to officiate.

Pre-financing of funerals can be accomplished by several methods. The following are included:

1. In some states, special burial or funeral insurance is available.

2. In most states, funeral homes can participate in special trust funds set up by individuals for the pre-financing of funeral costs.

Before taking steps to prearrange or pre-finance a funeral, consider these four factors:

1. The possible effect of your decision on survivors.

2. Logical planning now for what might not take place for many years.

3. The tentative nature of the plans.

4. The safety of any money paid in advance. Make sure any such money is protected under state trust laws or under insurance regulations. Most statutes provide that you can get all or most of it back at any time if you change plans.

Before prearranging a cemetery choice, be fairly sure this will be your final choice. An unwise purchase in advance may result in additional costs at the time of death.

Any document spelling out wishes to be followed, mandating a post-death activity, or indicating any financial arrangements should be in the possession of someone who most likely will survive your death. It should not be kept in a bank safety deposit box, because all post-death activities probably would be over long before the safety deposit box could be legally opened.

After her husband died without a will, my sister and her son, an experienced tax counselor, went to see their banker. At the conclusion of their conference, the banker said, "It looks to me like you're in good hands."

In the absence of steady survivors with such expertise, most of us could profit by making our own plans and preparing for an inevitable eventuality.

When we buy automobile insurance, we hope we never have an accident. When we buy home insurance, we hope we never have a fire. When we buy life insurance, we hope no one collects in the near future. And when we prearrange and pre-pay for a funeral, we hope we don't die right away. But just as surely as insurance brings peace of mind, so does the knowledge that you have made final arrangements.

We can now get on with our life, and our tour.

Chapter 11
Fairmont Freeway: Residential Section

I reserved this area until toward the end of our tour because it's the most fascinating part of Golden Acres.

In addition to those you've met already, here I'll introduce you to other neighbors who decided to continue living indefinitely. Unfortunately, we probably won't find many of them at home. They're out ministering, traveling, socializing, or working. But let's see who's here.

John and Thelma live here on the corner. No use looking for them. They're working at the college.

Mrs. Taylor lives here. She's probably at some kind of meeting. She belongs to several clubs.

As we approach the next house, we can hear Eva playing the piano and singing. Illness forced her to drop out of the church choir. But since she recuperated, she leads singing for her Sunday School class.

At church we heard Doctor Wheeler preach. He keeps busy in conventions and revivals. If you listen closely at their house, you can hear Mrs. Wheeler reading. She's a speech teacher. Shh! She's reading from Elizabeth Barrett Browning's poem:

"Grow old along with me, The best is yet to be."

Turning to us, she says, "I affirm this to be true; I have found it so." And her gracious manner and smile convince us that she means what she says.

Bradley and Marie live in the next house. They've recently returned from Switzerland, where he taught English for one semester. Bradley isn't at home. He's at his office at the college. Marie is making dolls to sell for gifts. She's at home.

Did you get a whiff of that turkey? Vernon and Lola must be preparing to cater another banquet. They won't have much time to talk to us.

I don't know his name, but this neighbor used to be an education specialist for the United States Government. Between church, family, neighborhood, and other group activities, he and his wife enjoy traveling. They've visited Europe, the Holy Land, Canada, and Mexico. They still find time for reading, writing, working in their greenhouse, and exercising. Don't expect to find them here.

Paul and Lillie are either traveling or writing. He has published some books since retirement. She writes articles.

Doctor Braswell is probably at the travel agency, where he servies as president. Mrs. Braswell may be busy preparing refreshments for her club meeting. If I'm correct, let's hope she'll give us a taste.

Listen! Do you hear music? Carl and Virgie live here. Carl is either giving a violin lesson or practicing for the church orchestra.

Lula and her mother live in this house. Lula hopes to travel later. For the present, however, she's taking care of her 95-year-old mother.

Fred and Laverne aren't at home either. He's probably holding a revival meeting somewhere. Or he may be at the college archives office where he works.

Charles drives cars for dealers. His wife arranges groups of drivers as needed. With a son and a son-in-law in the automobile business, they stay quite busy.

James Sanders preaches for various churches. During the week, he sometimes drives cars for dealers.

Milton and Edith live here. Milton works at the bank.

Do you hear that typewriter clattering at full speed? That's Joy, typing her novel. Between counseling sessions as a family therapist, she's taking writing courses at the university and working on a novel. Her husband works at the bank. In their "spare" time, they like to travel. I wish they had time to talk to us.

I must take you by to see Myrtle. She's a sweet, little 89 year old. Very alert. She's a bit humpy, but the sparkle in her eye and the radiance of her smile make her special.

She attends church almost every Sunday. At a club meeting a few months ago, she gave two readings from memory. She can tell some interesting stories of the old days.

Mr. Gardner had cancer surgery about twenty years ago. Since the operation was successful, he continues to get around. When I saw him at a banquet recently, he looked well.

Herman Johnson and his wife are involved in church and family activities. He works at his real estate office.

A nurse lives here. I don't know her name, but I know she likes to travel. When she's at home, she's gardening or working on arts and crafts. She complains of not having enough leisure time.

Henry is one of our church custodians. Believe me, it's a full-time job.

Duane and Wilma work part-time as church custodians. And Duane works some for the funeral home.

You'll notice beautiful lawns in this area. A lot of housewives enjoy gardening. And their husbands like to work in the yard. Some prefer to play indoor games or visit with friends. Some like tennis. Many of the men play golf. But few neglect their lawns.

Eating out is a favorite pastime, especially for the ladies. Restaurants attract seniors with discount prices. An overwhelming majority of customers in some cafeterias are senior adults.

I'm sorry so many of these neighbors either aren't at home or they're too busy to talk with us. But that's life in Golden Acres.

The next house stands apart because of the couple who live there. I want to introduce you to my retiree role models, Dr. and Mrs. Ray Jamison.

Only a few years older than I, they quit while they were ahead. And they have gauged their activities to make the most of retirement.

For years Doctor Jamison wrestled with problems inherent in a college presidency. Struggling to keep the institution alive and prosperous through periods of financial cuts, enrollment declines, and ownership changes, he looked forward to the serenity and freedom of retirement.

Periodic glimpses of this calm, relaxed gentleman, with a spring in his step and enthusiasm in his voice, convinced me that life begins at retirement—well, almost.

Between socializing, playing golf or tennis, traveling, or reading, the Jamisons are living it up. Both look great.

Oh, did I say "reading"? That reminds me. We'd better make a dash for the library before it closes.

Chapter 12
Golden Acres Public Library

We conclude our tour here because, hopefully, what you have learned so far has but served to whet your appetite for knowledge about our age group.

Our library contains various resources for learning about Golden Acres and its facilities.

First, I'll show you a list of resources I used for my information. Then I'll suggest other books and periodical titles you will find helpful. Finally, I'll mention various programs available to enhance senior-citizen living. A veritable gold mine of information awaits you.

In his essay *"Of Studies,"* Francis Bacon wrote:

Some books are to be tasted, others to be swallowed, and some few to be chewed, and digested; that is, some books are to be read only in parts; others to be read, but not curiously; and some few to be read wholly, and with diligence and attention.

If I may recommend one to be chewed and digested, it would be *The Silver Pages*, Senior Citizens Directory.

Notes: Chapter 2

[1] Arthur Fay Sueltz, *If I Should Die Before I Live* (Waco, Texas: Word Books, 1979), p.116.

[2] Robert N. Butler, *Why Survive? Being Old in America* (New York: Harper and Rowe, 1975), p.56.

[3] Gaston Foote, *Lamps Without Oil* (Montgomery, Alabama: The Paragon Press, 1944), pp.182-184.

[4] Ronald Gross et al., *The New Old: Struggling for Decent Aging* (Garden City, New York: Anchor Press/Doubleday, 1978), p.97.

[5] Robert C. Atchley, *The Social Forces in Later Life* 3rd. ed. (Belmont, California: Wadsworth Publishing Co., 1980), p.179.

[6] Atchley, p. 179.

[7] Atchley, p. 182.

[8] Mildred O. Hogstel, *Nursing Care of the Older Adult* (New York: John Wiley and Sons, 1981), p.42.

[9] Atchley, pp.172-174.

[10] "One in 5 Americans to Be Elderly By 2030, Census Bureau Predicts," *The Daily Oklahoman/Times*, 7 Sept. 1984, p.9.

[11] James J. Kilpatrick, "The Storm Ahead: Old Vs. Young" (editorial), *The Daily Oklahoman/Times*, 6 Oct. 1984.

[12] Butler, pp.6-11.

Notes: Chapter 4

[1] As You Like It, II. vii. 138-165.

[2] Earl Jabay, *Search for Identity*, p.13.

[3] Ferdie J. Deering, *The Daily Oklahoman*, 19 Nov. 1984, editorial page.

[4] Archibald MacLeish, "Who Precisely Do You Think You Are?" in *Interpreting Literature*, eds. K. L. Knickerbocker and H. Willard Reninger, 6th ed., p.839.

[5] "Hamlet," II. ii. 26-31.

[6] Jabay, Preface.

[7]Allene Jones, "Developmental Tasks of Later Middle Age and Old Age," in *Nursing Care of the Older Adult*, ed. Mildred O. Hogstel, p.34.
[8]Robert Butler, *Why Survive? Being Old in America*, p.72.
[9]Joyce Brothers, "First Person, Singular," *Mature Outlook* Nov.-Dec. 1985, p.62.
[10]Brothers, p.64.
[11]Brothers, p.66.
[12]Brothers, p.91-92.
[13]Butler, p.370.
[14]Mildred O. Hogstel, *Nursing Care of the Older Adult*, p. 71.
[15]Butler, p.16.
[16]Edwin Keister, Jr., "Getting a Jump on Living Longer," *50 Plus*, Sept. 1984, pp.15-20.
[17]Alex Comfort, "Aging: Real and Imaginary," in *The New Old: Struggling for Decent Aging*, eds. Ronald Gross, et al., p.75.
[18]Butler, p. 225.
[19]Comfort, p. 79.

Notes: Chapter 5

[1]Isadore Rossman, "Sexuality and Aging: an Internist's Perspective," in *Sexuality and Aging*, ed. Robert L. Solnick, p.70.
[2]Robert Kastenbaum, *Growing Old: Years of Fulfillment*, pp.82-83.
[3]Isadore Rubin, "The Sexless Older Years: A Socially Harmful Stereotype," in *Growing Old in America*, ed. Beth B. Hess, p.520.
[4]Rubin, p.521.
[5]Rossman, p.70.
[6]Joseph N. Bell, "Sex Therapy Can Save Your Marriage," *50 Plus*, Oct. 1984, p.29.
[7]Robert C. Atchley, *The Social Forces in Later Life*, p.350.

[8]Kastenbaum, p.83.
[9]Rossman, p.73.
[10]Bell, pp.29-33.
[11]"Sonnet 116."
[12]Arthur Fay Sueltz, *If I Should Die Before I Live*, p.37.

Notes: Chapter 7

[1]Paul Harvey, "Ethiopian 'Relocation' Really Another Holocaust," *The Daily Oklahoman*, March 19, 1986, Editorial page.

[2]Peter Weaver & Annette Buchanan, *What to Do with What You've Got*, Washington, D.C.: American Association of Retired Persons, pp.36-40.

[3]*Mature Outlook Newsletter*, Feb. 1986.

Notes on Chapter 9

[1]Hogstel, p.61.
[2]Hogstel, p.244.
[3]Kastenbaum, p.26.
[4]Peggy Kloster Yen, "Fat, Cholesterol, and a Healthy Older Heart," *Geriatric Nursing*, July/August, 1984, p.254.
[5]Yen, p.254.
[6]Yen, p.254.
[7]Yen, p.254.
[8]Yen, p.254.
[9]William A. Nolen, "The Checkup That May Save a Life—What Are You Waiting For?" *50 Plus*, August 1984, p.35.
[10]*The Weight Watchers Program*, Weight Watchers International, Inc., 1983, p.3.
[11]Butler, p.146.
[12]Bill Gale, "Talking About Walking," *50 Plus*, October 1984, pp.62-64.
[13]Provide Hospital, Portland, Oregon, in *Ostomy News*, Ostomy Association of Oklahoma City, Sept.1984.
[14]S. E. Sivertson, "Common Problems of Ambulatory

Geriatric Patients," *Postgraduate Medicine*, July 1984, p.86.

[15]Kastenbaum, p.23.

[16]Richard Rivlin, "Good Morning America," ABC, March 4, 1986.

[17]Monette Graves, "Physiologic Changes and Major Diseases in the Older Adult," in Hogstel, p.101.

[18]Edwin Keister, Jr., "Getting the Jump on Living Longer," *50 Plus*, Sept. 1984, p.16.

[19]Keister, pp.15-20.

[20]John Chancellor, "NBC Nightly News," Feb. 5, 1986.

[21]Keister, p.20.

[22]Robert W. Bermudes, *Conquering Cancer*, p.6.

[23]Bermudes, pp.13-15.

[24]"How Your Personality Affects Your Health," *Ostomy News*, Ostomy Association of Oklahoma City, Oct. 1985.

Bibliography

Atchley, Robert C. *The Social Forces in Later Life*. 3rd ed. Belmont, California: Wadsworth Publishing Co., 1980.

Bell, Joseph N. "Sex Therapy Can Save Your Marriage," *50 Plus*. Oct. 1984, pp.29-33.

Bermudes, Robert W. *Conquering Cancer*. Lima, Ohio: The C.S.S. Publishing Co., 1983.

Brothers, Joyce. "First Person, Singular," *Mature Outlook*. Nov.-Dec. 1985, pp.61-66; 90-92.

Butler, Robert N. *Why Survive? Being Old in America*. New York: Harper & Row, 1975.

Comfort, Alex. "Aging: Real and Imaginary," *The New Old: Struggling for Decent Aging*. Ronald Gross, et al. eds. Garden City, New York: Anchor Press/Doubleday, 1978.

Deering, Ferdie J. *The Daily Oklahoman*. 19 Nov. 1984, Editorial page.

Foote, Gaston. *Lamps Without Oil*. Montgomery, Ala.: The Paragon Press, 1944.

Gale, Bill. "Talking About Walking," *50 Plus*. Oct. 1984, pp.62-64.

Graves, Monette. "Physiologic Changes and Major Diseases in the Older Adult," *Nursing Care of the Older Adult*. Mildred O. Hogstel, ed. New York: John Wiley & Sons, 1981.

Gross, Ronald, *et al.* eds. *The New Old: Struggling for Decent Aging*. Garden City, N.Y.: Anchor Press/Doubleday, 1978.

Harvey, Paul. "Ethiopian 'Relocation' Really Another Holocaust." *The Daily Oklahoman*. March 19, 1986, Editorial page.

Hess, Beth B., ed. *Growing Old in America*. 2nd ed. New Brunswick: Transaction Books, 1980.

Hogstel, Mildred O. *Nursing Care of the Older Adult*. New York: John Wiley & Sons, 1981.

"How Your Personality Affects Your Health," *Ostomy News*. Ostomy Association of Oklahoma City, Oct. 1985.
Jabay, Earl. *Search for Identity*. Grand Rapids, MI.: Zondervan Publishing House, 1971.
Kastenbaum, Robert. *Growing Old: Years of Fulfillment*. New York: Harper & Row, 1979.
Keister, Edwin, Jr. "Getting a Jump on Living Longer," *50 Plus*. Sept. 1984, pp.15-20.
Kilpatrick, James J. "The Storm Ahead: Old Vs. Young." *The Daily Oklahoman*. Oct. 6, 1984. Editorial page.
MacLeish, Archibald, "Who Precisely Do You Think You Are?" *Interpreting Literature*. 6th ed. K. L. Knickerbocker and H. Willard Reninger, eds. New York: Holt, Rinehart, & Winston, 1978, pp.821-824.
Morrison, Malcolm H., ed. *Economics of Aging: The Future of Retirement*. New York: Van Nostrand Reinbold Co., 1982.
"One of 5 Americans to Be Elderly By 2030, Census Bureau Predicts." *The Daily Oklahoman and Times*. Sept. 7, 1984, p.9.
Rossman, Isadore. "Sexuality and Aging: An Internist's Perspective." *Sexuality and Aging*. Robert L. Solnick, ed. Los Angeles: The University of Southern California Press, 1978.
Rubin, Isadore. "The Sexless Older Years." *Growing Old in America*. Beth B. Hess. ed. 2nd ed. New Brunswick: Transaction Books, 1980.
Seymour, Eugene, ed. *Psychosocial Needs of the Aged*. Los Angeles: The University of Southern California Press, 1978.
Shakespeare, William. "As You Like It," II. vii.138-165. *The Complete Works of William Shakespeare*. 3rd ed. David Bevington, ed. Glenview, Ill.: Scott, Foresman & Co., 1980.
_____ "Hamlet," II.ii.26-31. *Interpreting Literature*. 6th ed. K. L. Knickerbocker and H. Willard Reninger, eds. New York: Holt, Rinehart, and Winston, 1978.
_____ "Sonnet 116." *The Complete Works of William*

Shakespeare. 3rd ed. David Bevington, ed. Glenview, Ill.: Scott, Foresman & Co., 1980.

Solnick, Robert L., ed. *Sexuality and Aging.* Los Angeles: The University of Southern California Press, 1978.

Sueltz, Arthur Fay. *If I Should Die Before I Live.* Waco, Texas: Word Books, 1979.

Take Charge of Your Money. A publication of the American Association of Retired Persons.

The Silver Pages, Senior Citizens Directory. St. Louis, Mo.: Southwestern Bell Media, Inc., 1985.

Weaver, Peter and Annette Buchanan. *What to Do with What You've Got.* An AARP Publication. Glenview, Ill.: Scott, Foresman and Co., 1984.

Yen, Peggy Kloster. "Fat, Cholesterol, and a Healthy Older Heart." *Geriatric Nursing.* July-August 1984, p. 254.

Suggested List of Periodicals

Dynamic Years, 215 Long Beach Blvd., Long Beach, CA 90802.

Mature Living, 127 9th Ave., N., Nashville, TN 37234.

Mature Years, 201 8th Ave., S., Nashville, TN 37202.

Modern Maturity, Publication of the AARP, 215 Long Beach Blvd., Long Beach, CA 90801.

Mature Outlook, Publications of Mature Outlook, Inc., 3701 W. Lake, Glenview, IL 60025.

Prime Times, Grote Deutsch & Co., Suite 120, 2802 International Ln., Madison, WI 53704.

Silver Circle, Publication of Home Savings of America/ Savings of America, Suite 2039, 4900 Rivergrade Rd., Irwindale, CA 91706.

New England Senior Citizen, A division of Prime National Publishing Corp., 470 Boston Post Rd., Weston, MA 02193.

Check your local Areawide Agency on Aging for pamphlets on all subjects dealing with senior citizens.

Those of you who really want to know what programs are available to retirees will be interested in the following pages of innovative programs

Innovative Programs

Virginia Fraser and Susan Thornton provided "An Inventory of Innovative Programs," compiled by the University Without Walls, at Loretto Heights College, in Denver, Colorado. This list was published in *The New Old: Struggling for Decent Aging*, Ronald Gross, et al. eds.

Communications

1. Senior's Radio Program

An hour-long talk show in San Diego—keeps elderly people informed and airs their opinions on issues and problems. KPBS-FM, San Diego, CA.

2. Televised Hearings on Aging

Ohio Commission on Aging enabled senior citizens to call a toll-free number to ask questions or state comments. Hearings are aired over twelve educational TV stations.

3. Combating Media Stereotypes

The National Council on Aging in Los Angeles provides a representative who attempts to convince the producer of the importance of changing the media attitude toward "the largest minority" in the United States. This representative provides information for programming.

The Gray Panthers senior citizens organization takes a more activist approach. It asks members to join its Media Watch. It provides forms and asks a watcher to write complaint letters or letters of commendation. Then it sends those letters and reports to TV producers.

4. Newspapers for Elders

There are many of them. For example, Colorado's *Senior Edition* and supplement *Colorado Old Times* deal with such issues as legislation, health care plans, state history, and nursing home scandals. These newspapers encourage reader contributions.

Another example is *The Phoenix*, Eugene, Oregon. It has "Features for Lively People 55 and Over," dealing with crime prevention, special cultural events and Social Security changes, and other issues.

5. Geriatrics Program Fair

Staged annually since 1974, the Norristown, PA., event provides senior citizens with information regarding programs and services, and puts agencies and professionals in the field of aging together on an informal basis, to compare programs and exchange ideas. The cost is minimal.

Education

1. Social work training for elders

The University of Washington in Seattle trains older people to be social workers.

2. Institute for Retired Professionals

NYC—a program run and taught by retirees. Dr. Hyman Hirsch, Director, Institute for Retired Professionals, New School for Social Research, 66 West 12th Street, New York, NY 10011.

3. The Alliance for Displaced Homemakers

This is a political advocacy group pushing laws to set up centers in every state to train displaced homemakers. The main emphasis is on self-confidence and how experience can be useful on the job. Mills College in Oakland, CA., has this program. There's one in Baltimore, Md., also.

Emotional Health

1. After-Care for Emotionally Frail Elders

The Texas Research Institute of Mental Sciences (TRIMS), of Houston, follows older patients dismissed from psychiatric institutions. It gets involved in medication regimes, transportation, and other community issues.

2. Grief Therapy Groups

Minneapolis Age and Opportunity Center, Inc., offers group support, involvement in problems with wills, probate, and taxes.

3. In-Home Mental Health Therapy

Seattle's King County provides the Community Home

Health Care facility.

4. SAGE—Senior Actualization and Growth Exploration

The purpose of this organization in Berkeley, CA., is to improve physical health and overcome elders' negative view of themselves. Biofeedback, art, breathing therapy, etc.—are part of this program.

5. Hospice for the Dying

The organization sends professionals and trained volunteers into the home, giving medical and emotional care to both families and patients. Pain control to make the patient as comfortable, active, and alert as possible is a major objective of the program. After the patient's death, the hospice visitor helps deal with the grieving family. Most large cities across the United States have a hospice program.

6. Sensitivity Course on Dying

Seattle Hospice offers a brief training program to educate professionals and volunteers so they can teach others how to deal with death and dying.

Many colleges and universities offer community service courses to help people deal with death and dying.

Employment

1. Job Placement Center Run by Elders

Experience, Inc., Palm Springs, CA., is run by seniors. They place people over 55 in both paid and volunteer jobs. These are mostly blue-collar jobs in hotels and private homes.

2. New Careers for Retired Law Professors

Hastings College, University of California at San Francisco, helps retired law professors to start new careers.

3. Unusual Job Opportunities

Part-time jobs with the federal government are available.

a. The National Weather Service offers both paid and volunteer job opportunities. Needs include cooperative weather observers and second order station observers.

First order station observers record maximum and minimum temperatures and rainfall each day, fill out forms, and send in a monthly report. The Weather Service trains second order station observers and installs the instruments at their homes to enable them to perform the same duties.
  b. Census takers draw an hourly wage and mileage.
  c. The United States Forest Service Campground Program operates at a dozen National Forests across the U.S. In this program, volunteer hosts live free for the season in small trailers set up in campgrounds. The host may do light cleaning or stock bathrooms with paper supplies. But one major consideration is the fact that the host's presence discourages vandalism.

If interested in any of these government jobs, you can contact (a) your nearest Weather Service, Forecast Office, Substation, Network Specialist; (b) your nearest regional Census Bureau office; (c) U.S. Forest Service, Agriculture South Building, 12th and Independence Ave., S.W., Washington, D.C. 20250.

Food and Nutrition

1. Grocery Shopping Service
Sacramento Elderly Nutrition Program, in Sacramento, CA., offers this service.
2. Mobile Mini-Market
This is a food advisory service, offered in Sacramento.
3. Brown Bag Food Programs
Volunteer senior citizens in this program ask produce growers to donate culls. Other older volunteers sort and bag the produce and staff distribution centers in the area. Volunteers may pick crops for which market conditions aren't right. This method saves growers labor costs and provides senior citizens with high-quality food, otherwise left to rot.
4. Space Age Meals-on-Wheels or by Mail
In Houston, Texas, this program delivers in person or by mail frozen astronaut meals to senior citizens.

Housing and Convalescent Care

1. Respite Care
Private homes or group centers are available to give family members a chance for a vacation or rest.

2. Do-It-Yourself Energy Conservation
A Colorado program—Domestic Technology Institute—gave solar energy workshops for senior citizens. They learned how to build passive solar panels covering 64 sq. ft. Fans blow solar-heated air into the house, saving up to 50% of energy costs.

Some built solar-heated greenhouses attached to their homes, thus cutting both food and heating costs.

The Community Action Agency of Laramie County, Cheyenne, WY., asked the Institute to offer a workshop on building community greenhouses fueled by a methane gas digester. Senior citizen volunteers built greenhouses and raised food for themselves and some to sell.

For workshop information: Contact Andree Dunn, Development Technology Institute, Box 2043, Evergreen, CO 80439.

For greenhouse information: Contact Al Duran, Executive Director, Community Action Program, Suite 400, Bell Bldg., Cheyenne, WY 82001.

3. Nursing Home Residents' Councils
Gray Panthers urge residents' councils for every nursing home. They try to convince residents that this is their home and that the employees—from doctor on down—are working for the residents.

The Gray Panthers helped set one up at Post Street Convalescent Hospital in San Francisco. Patients meet monthly for information on various health problems. They can complain to representatives from various hospital departments. If their problems can't be solved, the staff must explain why they can't.

Mary Godfrey, Activities Director, Post Street Convalescent Hospital, 2130 Post Street, San Francisco, CA 94115, is the contact person.

4. An Intergenerational Housing Effort

Ladies of Charity of the United States—Roman Catholic—Washington, D.C., encourages senior citizens to take in student roomers. These are closely screened by volunteers or priests. Many are foreign students. This arrangement helps both parties financially.

5. Home Repair Services

New Orleans has a Repairs on Wheels program. Volunteers make minor repairs on homes owned by senior citizens.

Skills Exchange of Arapahoe County, CO., wasn't too successful because some senior citizens couldn't exchange skills. Local service clubs ended up doing most of the repairs.

6. Tax Work-Off Program

Hartford, Connecticut, allowed senior citizens to perform work, ranging from unskilled to clerical to data processing in exchange for tax credits.

The purpose of Golden Acres Educational Tours is to enable you to thrive, as well as survive, after 55. To answer affirmatively the question "If I retire shall I live again?" What you've learned on this tour should help you really live your final years productively.

Dr. Lloyd Ogilvie, Pastor of Hollywood Presbyterian Church, gives some valuable hints. He says that some people affirm: "For me, to live is to be a banker" (or whatever their profession or occupation may be). But the Apostle Paul declared: "For to me to live *is* Christ..." (Phil. 1:21).

To really live, we do well to pray with Doctor Ogilvie:

"Lord, what you give me
  the Vision to Conceive,
    and the Power to Believe,
      I completely Trust You to help me to Achieve,
      All that You have Dreamed for me."

Printed in the United States
1537000001B/620